OBSTETRIC ULTRASOUND

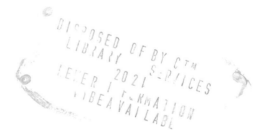

To
Ben, Megan and Emma,
perhaps the best reasons for teaching ultrasound

For Churchill Livingstone:

Publisher: Mary Law
Editorial Co-ordination: Editorial Resources Unit
   Copy Editor: Neil Pakenham-Walsh
   Indexer: Nina Boyd
Production Controller: Nancy Henry
Design: Design Resources Unit
Sales Promotion Executive: Hilary Brown

OBSTETRIC ULTRASOUND:
HOW, WHY AND WHEN

Patricia Chudleigh
BSc DMU
Research Assistant,
Department of Obstetric Ultrasound,
King's College Hospital,
London

J. Malcolm Pearce
MD FRCS FRCOG
Senior Lecturer,
Department of Obstetrics and Gynaecology,
St George's Hospital Medical School,
London

Foreword by
Stuart Campbell
MB ChB FRCOG
Professor and Head, Department of
Obstetrics and Gynaecology,
King's College Hospital, London

SECOND EDITION

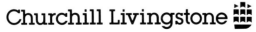

EDINBURGH LONDON MADRID MELBOURNE NEW YORK AND TOKYO 1992

CHURCHILL LIVINGSTONE
Medical Division of Longman Group UK Limited

Distributed in the United States of America by Churchill Livingstone Inc.,
650 Avenue of the Americas New York, N.Y. 10011, and by associated companies, branches
and representatives throughout the world.

First edition 1986
Second edition 1992
  Reprinted 1993

ISBN 0-443-04207-1

British Library Cataloguing in Publication Data
A catalogue record for this book is available from the British Library.

Library of Congress Cataloging in Publication Data
Chudleigh, Patricia.
    Obstetric ultrasound: how, why, and when/Patricia Chudleigh, J.
  Malcolm Pearee; foreword by Stuart Campbell. — 2nd ed.
      p.   cm.
    Includes bibliographical references and index.
    ISBN 0-443-04207-1
    1. Ultrasonics in obstetrics.   I. Pearce, J. Malcolm (John
  Malcolm)
    [DNLM: 1. Pregnancy Complications — diagnosis.   2. Prenatal
  Diagnosis — methods.   3. Ultrasonography — in pregnancy. WQ 209
  C559o]
  RG527.5.U48C48   1992
  618.2′2 — dc20
  DNLM/DLC
  for Library of Congress   91-19234

The
publisher's
policy is to use
paper manufactured
from sustainable forests

Produced by Longman Singapore Publishers (Pte) Ltd
Printed in Singapore

FOREWORD

This book is written by two of the most accomplished practitioners in the field of obstetric scanning. Malcolm Pearce and Patricia Chudleigh developed their skills in the largest high risk obstetric ultrasound clinic in the UK and they were deeply involved in the running of the advanced obstetric ultrasound course at King's College Hospital where they learned to communicate their expertise. Since writing the first edition of this book, Malcolm Pearce has set up a major fetal medicine centre at St George's Hospital and has continued his interest in Doppler ultrasound, while Patricia Chudleigh has considerably expanded her involvement in teaching and research work including co-ordinating multicentre studies on fetal choroid plexus cysts and renal pelvic dilatation.

The first edition has become a standard textbook for obstetric scanning. The present volume consolidates the aims of the first edition which is to provide a comprehensive account of ultrasound techniques and their clinical applications in a clear and concise manner. The new edition expands on this to include chapters on the rapidly developing areas of ultrasound diagnosis such as Doppler ultrasound and transvaginal sonography.

This book is a superb introduction to anyone who wishes to become involved in one of the most exciting and rewarding new areas of medicine.

S.C.

PREFACE
TO THE SECOND EDITION

The past 5 years have witnessed major advances in ultrasound imaging. The development of high frequency transvaginal probes has revolutionised follicular tracking and has greatly improved the monitoring of the first trimester of pregnancy. The resolution of real-time apparatus is now such that the diagnosis of subtle fetal abnormalities is well within the reach of the ultrasonographer working in a routine setting. Doppler ultrasound has become established as a means of monitoring the small-for-gestational-age fetus. By its frequent use we have realised that only a few small-for-gestational-age fetuses are pathological. This has meant less interference in normal pregnancies but more appropriately timed intervention for the fetus in genuine trouble. Invasive procedures have increased in type and frequency and whilst most are performed by obstetricians the ultrasonographer is often required to perform the imaging.

These improvements have not been without problems. Many minor abnormalities are now being detected, the significance of which is not truly known. Uninformed and unsympathetic explanations can lead to unnecessary maternal anxiety. Use of Doppler ultrasound in situations where there is little or no supporting evidence for its use has led to false reassurance with disastrous outcomes. We hope that the second edition of our text will fulfil the same aims as the first edition but will also address the new techniques in a rational fashion. This edition not only describes how to obtain the required images but also gives practical guidelines on the interpretation of the findings. The suggestions in the text are a distillate of those we both use in our own practice, and as such have grown from many years of working in teaching centres with high referral rates. We believe that those who follow the advice given, be they clinicians or technicians, will reassure the woman with a normal pregnancy. Management of women with an abnormal pregnancy now commonly involves a team approach with ultrasonographers, obstetricians, paediatric surgeons, neonatologists and geneticists but the guidelines we have given should allow the ultrasonographer to talk to the women in an informative fashion before making arrangements for further referral.

London, 1992   P.C.
                                                                    J.M.P.

CONTENTS

CHAPTER ONE
Preparing to scan

In order to obtain maximum information from any ultrasound examination the following three points should be observed:

1. The ultrasound equipment should be suited to the required examination and should be functioning correctly
2. The patient should be properly prepared
3. You, as the operator, should be confident in your abilities to perform the examination.

THE ULTRASOUND EQUIPMENT: COMPONENTS AND THEIR USES

Real-time equipment currently available varies greatly in size, shape and complexity, but will contain six basic components:

- The probe, in which the transducer is housed
- A scan converter and monitor
- A control panel
- A freeze frame
- Measuring facilities
- A means of taking hard copy.

The probe

This refers to the piece of equipment in which the transducer, (or transducers) is mounted. The transducer is a piezoelectric crystal(s) which, when activated electronically, produces pulses of sound at very high frequencies — this is known as ultrasound. The crystal can also work in reverse in that it can convert the echoes returning from the body into electrical signals from which the ultrasound images are made up.

In practice, however, the terms probe and transducer are used interchangeably. The probe may be either a conventional type used externally or an intracavity type such as that used transvaginally. There are two broad types of transducer: linear and sector. These terms refer to the way in which the crystal or crystals are arranged and manipulated to produce an image, and they may be further subdivided into:

a. Linear — flat-faced linear, curvilinear or convex sector, phased array and annular array
b. Sector — mechanical, wobbler or electrical.

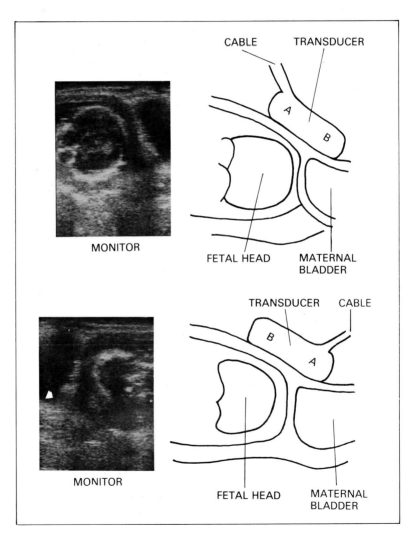

Fig. 1.1 Diagram to demonstrate that one end of the transducer always relates to the same side of the screen. The end of the transducer labelled 'A' relates to the left side of the screen regardless of the orientation on the maternal abdomen.

The image field produced by the flat-faced linear transducer is rectangular while all the others are sector in shape.

Irrespective of its type, the probe is one of the most expensive and delicate parts of the equipment. It is easily damaged if knocked or dropped and so should always be replaced in its housing when not in use.

The left–right display of information on the ultrasound monitor is determined by the probe. One side of the probe (see point A in Fig. 1.1) always relates to one side of the ultrasound monitor. This relationship is constant however the probe is positioned (the exception being when the left–right invert control is used — see below). When performing longitudinal scans of the pelvis using the abdominal method (as opposed to the transvaginal method) the bladder is conventionally shown on the right of the image on the ultrasound monitor (see Fig. 1.1). The eccentric cable insertion in many linear and curvilinear probes is a useful guide to orientation.

Exactly the same principles apply with the other types of probe, although their symmetrical shape and smaller size often makes orientation difficult initially. The probe will generally have a mark, notch or other means of identification on one side which helps distinguish longitudinal from transverse, before experience takes over!

Failure to understand these principles can easily lead to confusion when localising the placenta or diagnosing fetal lie. An innocuous fundal placenta may be diagnosed as placenta praevia and a cephalic

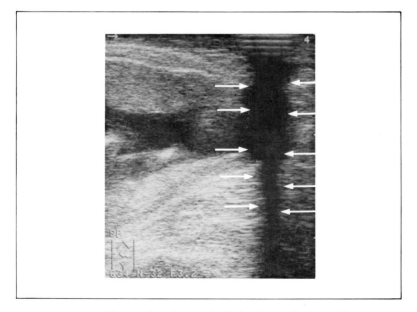

Fig. 1.2 Diagram to illustrate how the acoustic shadow (arrowed) produced by a finger introduced under one end of the transducer helps to orientate the scan.

presentation may be mistaken for a breech if the transducer orientation is not appreciated.

When scanning in transverse or oblique planes the relationship between one end of the transducer (point A) and one side of the screen remains. A rather unscientific, but easy method of confirming left and right is to run a finger under one end of the transducer. The shadow seen on the monitor relates to the position of the finger (Fig. 1.2).

The left–right invert control, as its name suggests, reverses this carefully elucidated orientation. Unless you are really familiar with ultrasound orientation you should always scan with this control in one position.

At the present time there is no convention for orientation when using transvaginal imaging. Confusingly, many machines reverse the orientation when switching from the abdominal probe to the transvaginal probe. A detailed description of orientation with vaginal probes will be found in Chapter 2.

The scan converter and monitor (see also Ch. 15)

Ideally there should be two monitors: a monitor for the operator to view the image and a monitor from which hard copy can be made. A separate viewing monitor is preferable as a larger screen is more restful to look at over long periods of time and is easier for the woman to see. It also allows individual preferences of image brightness and contrast to be catered for without affecting the settings (and gamma control) required for hard copy.

The control panel

In general, the fewer the controls, the better and the more consistent are the images obtained. Sound, be it audible or ultrasound, can be regulated by a volume control which, in the case of ultrasound, is known as a gain control. In simple terms, the more sound received by the transducer the brighter the image. The amount of sound entering the patient is determined by the overall gain control, and this should be kept as low as possible. The amplification of the returning echoes is known as time-gain compensation (TGC — see Ch. 16). The controls for this may simply be labelled as near and far gain, each affecting the upper or lower half of the screen respectively. Alternatively, the machine may have a series of sliders that control slices (usually about 2 cm in depth) of the image.

The gain control settings are crucial in the quality of the image displayed. Too little gain produces a very dark image (Fig. 1.3a) whilst too much gain produces too bright an image (Fig. 1.3b) and also exposes the patient to an unnecessarily high dose of ultrasound. Inappropriate settings of the TGC will produce dark and/or light bands

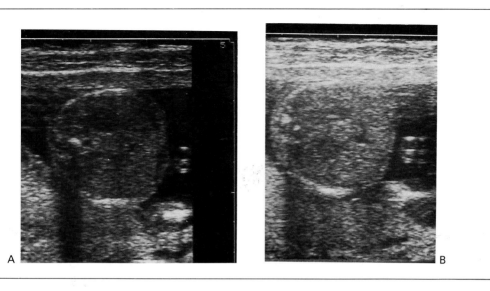

Fig. 1.3 Incorrect gain settings. (a) Too little gain. (b) Too much gain. Compare these with Figure 1.4a, which has the correct gain control settings. Notice how much more detail is seen from the structures within the fetal abdomen.

within the image. The correct gain settings produce the image shown in Figure 1.4(a).

Fetal structures can be identified more easily and the margin of error in measurement is less when a magnified image is used. It is good practice to always scan and record images using as magnified an image as is comfortably possible.

Most equipment now offers a rejection (or suppression) control. This suppresses noise electronically but it also suppresses low level echoes that are essential in identifying fetal anatomy. It is usually, therefore, set to its minimum value.

Some equipment also offers pre- and post-processing (see Ch. 16). Pre-processing is of limited use in general obstetrics, although using it to produce an image with more contrast is useful in performing follicular and early pregnancy examinations.

Time gain controls (depth gain controls) and their setting are explained in Chapter 15.

Freeze frame control

This is essential for taking measurements and for making hard copy. The position of the control varies. It may be an integral part of the transducer casing, positioned on the control panel or, most conveniently, a foot switch.

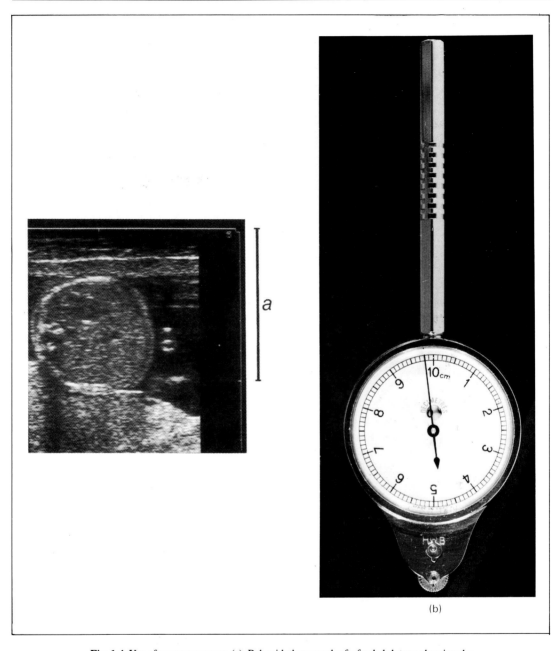

Fig. 1.4 Use of a map measurer. (a) Polaroid photograph of a fetal abdomen showing the correct gain control settings. (b) Map measurer. As the Polaroid image is less than life-size, the distance between the cm markers along the top and right edges is reduced. Measuring the distance between five of these marks produces the conversion factor a, which is 4 cm in this picture. The outline of the abdominal circumference is measured with a map measurer and produces the result b, which is 9.8 cm in this picture. The life-size abdominal circumference c, is obtained as follows:

$c = 9.8 \times 5/4 = 12.25$ cm

On-screen measurement

Most machines provide facilities for linear, circumference and area measurements. These may be displayed alone or together with an interpretation of, for example, gestational age or fetal weight. The gestational age given will vary depending upon the charts programmed into the machine. We recommend that the sonographer interprets the measurements from each examination himself rather than relying exclusively on the machine. For example, interpreting measurements made in late pregnancy in terms of gestational age is wrong (see Ch. 11).

The velocity of the caliper system (see Ch. 16) is set by the manufacturer and must be known for each machine. Most machines have caliper system velocities set at 1540 m/s, although velocities of 1600 m/s or 1580 m/s are also used. The majority of caliper systems are of the joystick or rollerball types. As with all techniques, on-screen measuring requires expertise and it is therefore good practice to take several (we suggest three) measurements of any parameter to ensure accuracy. Linear measurements should be reproducible to within 1 mm, and circumference measurements to within 3 mm.

Recording systems

The majority of machines now have comprehensive on-screen measuring facilities allowing a quick and cheap method of obtaining circumference and area measurements. Video facilities, the Polaroid camera attachment or the thermal imager are necessary only for making a permanent record of interesting or abnormal images. Hopefully, most sonographers will never have to use the old-fashioned techniques of calculating circumference values using hard copy and a map measurer, but we have included this technique for completeness.

When using Polaroid photographs for measurement, two factors are important:

- The image is square, i.e. a set distance along the horizontal (x-axis) is equal to that along the vertical (y-axis)
- The conversion factor for the image size can be calculated.

Every machine displays 1 cm markers superimposed on every image. After taking a blank Polaroid photograph, measure the distance between ten of these markers both horizontally and vertically using a ruler. If the value is the same along both axes then the image is square. If the distance differs, then alter the horizontal or vertical controls of the monitor until the distance along both axes is identical.

The distance between five markers would measure 5 cm if the camera produced life-size images. As it does not, this distance a provides the conversion factor when calculating non-linear measurements. If the circumference measurement obtained using the map measurer is b, then the life-size value c can be calculated as below:

c (cm) $= b$ (cm) $\times 10 / a$ (cm)

See Figure 1.4 for a worked example.

The sensitivity of Polaroid film is such that small alterations in camera settings (shutter speed or aperture) or on the monitor (brightness or contrast) will produce large differences in the quality of the Polaroid photograph. Ideally, the camera controls and those of the machine should be set when the machine is installed. Once ideal settings have been obtained it is advisable to cover the controls with adhesive tape to discourage over-keen colleagues from fiddling with them. Apparent deterioration in the quality of the photographs taken is usually due to poor gain settings or insufficient coupling gel.

Polaroid film is very temperature sensitive, so ensure your films are always stored at a constant, cool temperature.

THE PATIENT

The woman should be given the opportunity to change into a gown prior to being scanned, to avoid the inconvenience and embarrassment of gel-stained clothing. The woman should lie on the examination couch such that she is able to see the screen easily. Most scans are performed with the woman supine or with her head slightly raised. However, in later pregnancy many women feel dizzy in this position (the supine hypotension syndrome) and it may be necessary for her to be tilted to one side. This is easily achieved by placing a pillow under one of the buttocks. If the woman's legs are covered with a clean sheet she will feel less embarrassed. This is just as important when performing vaginal examinations as abdominal examinations. The woman will feel less vulnerable and less embarrassed by this courtesy on behalf of the operator.

When performing an abdominal scan the woman should be uncovered just sufficiently to allow the examination to be performed. This will always include the first inch of the area covered by her pubic hair and will extend far enough upwards to allow the fundus of the uterus to be visualised. It is thoughtful to protect her underwear by tucking paper towels into the top of her knickers.

A full bladder is the only prerequisite for an abdominal ultrasound examination. This is usually only necessary in non-pregnant women those of less than 12 weeks gestation or in women in whom a low-lying placenta is suspected. In order to get the bladder full enough for the examination the woman should be asked to drink two pints of water or squash one hour before attending the department. She should not empty her bladder until after the scan is completed. She should be made to understand that one cup of coffee on the way to the department is inadequate and will result in a long wait. When the bladder is overfull and the woman is in obvious discomfort, partial bladder emptying is the best solution. Sufficient urine will usually be retained to make a successful examination possible.

Scanning transvaginally naturally requires the woman to remove all her lower clothing. Ideally, she should be positioned on a gynaecological couch, with her legs supported by low stirrups, thus allowing maximum ease of access to the pelvic organs. This is especially important when examining the ovaries and adnexae. However, an adequate improvisation is to place two chairs at one end of the examination table. The woman lies on the table with her bottom as near to the end of the table as possible and rests her feet on the two chairs.

When scanning transvaginally an empty bladder is a prerequisite. Send the woman to the toilet before beginning a transvaginal examination as even a small amount of urine in the bladder can push the important part of the uterus below, that is posterior to, and therefore out of the field of view of, this high frequency transducer.

The transvaginal probe should be kept immersed in a sterilising fluid, e.g. Cidex, when not in use. If the probe cannot be immersed then it should be sprayed with a hard surface disinfectant. We suggest the following regime when preparing the transvaginal transducer. Apply a small amount of gel to the transducer tip and cover the tip and shaft of the probe with a (non-spermicidal) condom. Apply a small amount of gel, or KY jelly, to the covered probe to allow easier insertion into the vagina.

THE OPERATOR

It is immaterial whether you are normally left- or right-handed as to which hand is 'better' for holding the transducer. It is important that the transducer is always held in the hand nearer the woman as this prevents you tying yourself in knots as you scan or dropping the transducer. It is a matter of individual or departmental preference as to whether the ultrasound machine is positioned to the left or the right of the examination couch. However, the majority of manufacturers work on the right-handed scanning technique and position the cables appropriately.

Transvaginal scanning generally requires a different arrangement of operator and machine. Ensure you are positioned in front of the perineum with the ultrasound machine close enough to operate the controls easily with your non-scanning hand. If the machine is too far away you will jar the vagina with the probe as you stretch forward or sideways to reach the controls.

Do ensure the woman can see the monitor easily when you are

scanning her transvaginally. Initially, many women find this method of examination embarrassing. Being able to watch the images on the monitor will often help her to relax and distract her from what you are doing to her.

Manual dexterity with either technique will be lacking initially, but rapidly improves with practice. Ensure that you are sitting comfortably and at the right height. If the stool is too low, you will quickly develop an aching shoulder; if too high, your foot will ache from continuously trying to reach the foot switches. Try to think of the probe as an extension of your arm rather than a foreign object, and do not grip it fiercely as this will also produce a painful arm and shoulder.

Always keep your foot resting on the freeze frame foot switch so that you can instantly freeze an image if necessary. You will lose many potentially 'perfect' images if you have to go searching for the foot switch.

There are many proprietary brands of coupling medium available, the variations being in viscosity, colour and price. All fulfil the same function of providing an air-free interface between the transducer and the body. Ultrasound gel at room temperature feels very cold so try to ensure the gel is warmed before starting an examination. It is now possible to purchase electric bottle warmers designed specifically for the ultrasound market. A baby's bottle warmer or a bowl of hot water, regularly replenished, are cheaper, although potentially more dangerous, alternatives. Apply the gel sparingly but remember that you will need more gel in the areas of skin covered with hair.

TRANSDUCER MOVEMENTS

There are only a limited number of ways in which the transducer can be manipulated. If you understand what each of these movements achieves you will quickly learn how to obtain the correct sections. You will also understand how to move from a less than ideal section to the perfect section and when this is difficult, for example due to fetal position, you will not waste time trying to achieve the impossible. Transvaginal scanning involves different movements from those used abdominally.

The abdominal probe

There are four possible movements of this probe:

1. *Sliding.* By holding the probe longitudinally and sliding it from side to side across the abdomen you change the level of the sagittal section. If the probe is held transversely and slid up and down, the level of the transverse section obtained is altered. With the probe still held transversely it can be slid across the woman's abdomen, a manoeuvre

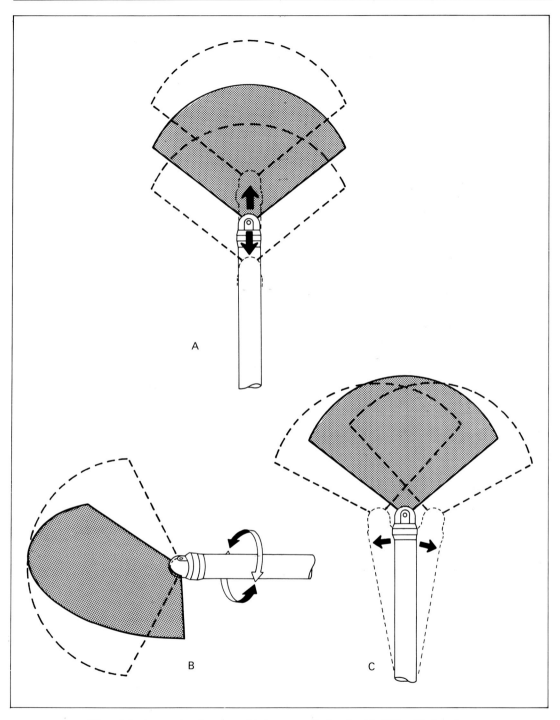

Fig. 1.5 Basic scanning directions with the transvaginal probe. (a) Sliding (b) Rotation
(c) Panning

that is useful for keeping the image under inspection in the centre of the screen.

2. *Rotating*. This term describes rotation of the probe about a fixed point. Its main use is that it allows a longitudinal section to be obtained from a transverse section of an organ (or vice versa) whilst keeping the organ in view.

3. *Angling*. This describes an alteration of the angle of the probe relative to the skin surface. Its main use is for obtaining correct sections from slightly oblique views.

4. *Dipping*. This describes pushing one end of the transducer into the maternal abdomen. It is uncomfortable, so should be done as gently as possible. Its main use is to bring structures of interest to lie at right angles to the sound beam.

The vaginal probe (see Fig. 1.5)

Four movements are also possible with this probe, but they are limited by the available space within the vagina. All movements of transvaginal probes should be carried out slowly and gently. It is important to learn how to insert the probe on your machine so that you obtain a true sagittal section.

1. *Sliding*. This describes the movement of the probe along the length of the vagina. As vaginal probes have a small field of view, sliding up and down the vagina is necessary to image the whole pelvis.

2. *Rotating*. This describes a circular movement of the handle of the probe. Rotating the probe through 90° from the position required for a true sagittal section gives a coronal view of the pelvis. Other degrees of rotation are usually necessary to image pelvic organs.

3. *Rocking*. This describes movement of the handle of the probe in an anteroposterior plane such that the tip of the probe moves in the opposite direction. This moves the field of view through a maximum arc of 60°. Further movement is limited by the woman's perineum posteriorly and her urethra anteriorly. The main use of this movement is in an attempt to image the true longitudinal section of the uterus when its position is not axial.

4. *Panning*. This is a photographic term which describes movement of the handle of the probe in a horizontal plane such that the tip of the probe moves in an opposite direction. This moves the field of view through a maximum arc of about 130°.

A gentle touch is one well worth developing whether scanning abdominally or transvaginally. The lightest pressure of the probe on the abdomen is sufficient to produce the majority of images. Digging the probe into the woman rarely improves the image quality and only causes unnecessary discomfort, especially if the woman has a full bladder.

Finally, a relaxed and informal atmosphere will give the woman confidence not only in your scanning abilities but also to ask any questions which she may feel are important. The majority of obstetric examinations should be pleasant, painless and reassuring to the woman, but the benefits, be they medical or emotional, are directly dependent upon the quality of operator input.

CHAPTER TWO
Ultrasound appearances of the normal pelvis

Scanning the non-pregnant or early pregnant pelvis can be performed using abdominal or transvaginal probes. Unfortunately, for the beginner, the two techniques are very different. This simple fact can leave even the most experienced operator acutely depressed when attempting a transvaginal examination for the first time. Irrespective of the method, once you have learnt how to orientate the probe to obtain longitudinal (sagittal) and cross-sectional views of the pelvis, the examination becomes easy.

SCANNING THE UTERUS

The uterus lies centrally within the pelvis, posterior to the bladder and cephalad to the vagina (Fig. 2.1). It is usually anteverted and rotated slightly to the right (dextrorotated).

Abdominal method

To perform a pelvic ultrasound examination using the abdominal route, the woman must have a full bladder. This has three effects: firstly, it pushes the uterus out of the pelvis, thus removing it from the acoustic shadow caused by the symphysis pubis; secondly, it provides an acoustic window through which the pelvic organs can be visualised; and thirdly, it displaces the bowel superiorly, so preventing gas from the bowel scattering the ultrasound beam.

In order to scan the nooks and crannies of the pelvis a transducer with a small area of contact is needed. This is most commonly a sector scanner, but phased array, annular array and small convex probes (curvilinear) are also appropriate. Although images of the pelvis can be obtained with the linear and curvilinear probes designed for obstetric

14

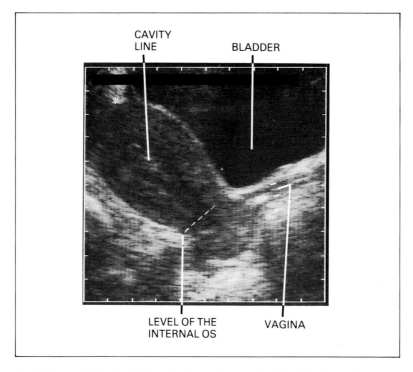

Fig. 2.1 Longitudinal (sagittal) section through a normal pelvis. Note the scan is orientated such that the bladder is on the right of the image. The cursor (white asterisk) indicates the uterine fundus.

use, their size makes a complete examination difficult and they may produce lateral artifacts (see Ch. 3).

Place the probe in the midline of the woman to obtain a longitudinal section with the bladder on the right of the screen. The vagina is usually immediately visualised as three bright parallel lines posterior to the bladder (Fig. 2.1). If only the lower part of the uterus is seen, rotate the probe slightly towards the right side of the woman, to compensate for the dextrorotation of the uterus.

In true longitudinal section the uterus demonstrates low level homogeneous echoes with a centrally placed strong linear echo from the cavity line (Fig. 2.1). This represents the interface between the adjacent endometrial surfaces of the uterus. In addition the section should clearly demonstrate the uterine fundus and will usually demonstrate the upper part of the vagina (Fig. 2.1).

The cervix is often difficult to define in non-pregnant women because of the angle at which the cervical canal lies relative to the sound beam. This remains a problem irrespective of whether the uterus is anteverted or retroverted. The position of the internal os can be gauged as it lies directly beneath the point at which the posterior wall of the bladder appears to change direction (Fig. 2.1). This change in direction occurs because the lower part of the bladder (the trigone) is fixed to the cervix and cannot change position as the bladder fills.

Cross-sectional views of the uterus are obtained by rotating the probe through 90° whilst keeping the cavity line in view. Sliding the probe up and down the abdomen will produce transverse sections of the uterus from cervix to fundus.

Problems

The fundus of the uterus will not be visualised unless the bladder is filled sufficiently to cover it.

A retroverted uterus occurs in about a third of women and is more common after pregnancy. The uterine fundus and the upper part of the cavity line may not be visualised in this situation because it is impossible to direct the ultrasound beam at right angles to them. Further filling of the bladder is of little help except to displace the bowel which lies between the bladder and the uterus. If a transvaginal probe is not available then little can be done in this situation except to ask a gynaecologist to antevert the uterus vaginally whilst the woman is being scanned. There is often obvious reluctance to perform vaginal examinations in the ultrasound department but it should be done if the situation is urgent. For example, if an ectopic pregnancy is suspected clinically, the demonstration of an intrauterine gestation sac with ultrasound will effectively exclude an ectopic gestation.

By 8 weeks gestation the uterine contents should always be visible, even with a steeply retroverted uterus, because the fluid within the gestation sac provides an easily recognisable echo free space. However, make sure you are certain this is a gestation sac and not fluid in the uterine cavity (pseudo-gestation sac) accompanying an ectopic pregnancy (see Ch. 4).

Transvaginal method

Preparation for transvaginal examination is described in Chapter 1. Hold the prepared probe with the mark or guide positioned to produce a longitudinal view of the pelvis and insert it gently into the vagina. The uterus will usually be visualised by panning the tip of the probe slightly towards the woman's right shoulder (to compensate for dextrorotation) and then rocking the handle posteriorly towards the perineum. By gently panning the probe to left and right the optimal longitudinal view of the uterine cavity will be obtained (Fig. 2.2). Do not rotate the probe simultaneously with panning as this will alter your orientation. In order to ensure that the view is truly longitudinal the entire length of the cavity line should be visualised as for the abdominal approach.

Transverse views of the uterus are more difficult to obtain and

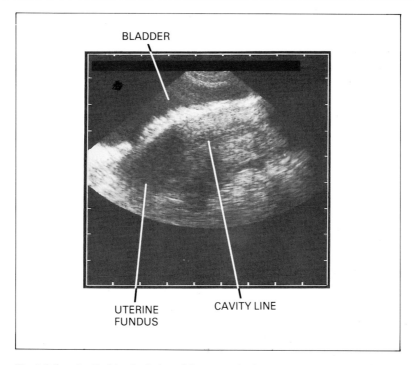

BLADDER

UTERINE
FUNDUS

CAVITY LINE

Fig. 2.2 Longitudinal (sagittal) view of the uterus obtained by means of a transvaginal probe. Much less of the pelvis is visualised because of the small field of view. There is still some urine in the bladder, which is visualised superiorly to an anteverted uterus.

interpret. Figure 2.3 illustrates the sections of the uterus that can be obtained. It is important to appreciate that the position and the degree of flexion of the uterus relative to the vagina determine the views obtained when the probe (or the beam) is rotated through 90° from a sagittal to a coronal section. For this reason cross-sectional views obtained by means of a vaginal probe are not comparable with those obtained abdominally.

The major advantage of the transvaginal probe is that its proximity to the pelvic organs allows a higher frequency transducer (usually 6–7.5 MHz) to be used. This increases the resolution but reduces the field of view such that forming a mental image of the entire pelvis is more difficult.

Problems

Visualising a retroverted uterus is far less problematic with this method. However, the vaginal diameter may limit posterior rocking movements so as to prevent visualisation of the fundus in a steeply retroverted uterus. Lack of sound penetration, due to the high

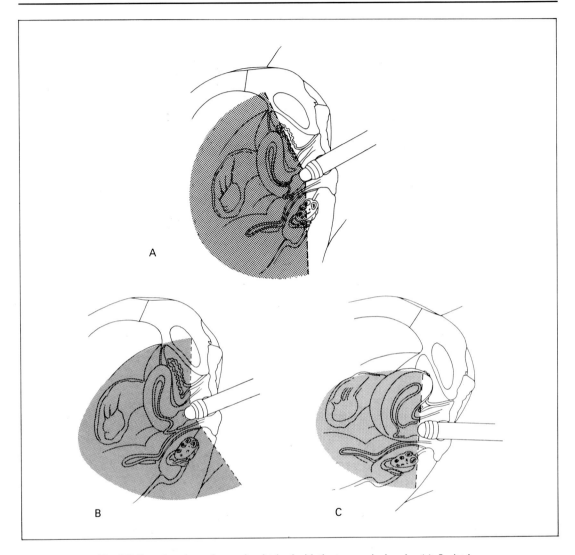

Fig. 2.3 Scanning planes that can be obtained with the transvaginal probe. (a) Sagittal or vertical plane. (b) Coronal or horizontal plane. (c) Because the perineum prevents downward depression of the probe, an oblique view of the uterine fundus is obtained when the uterus is very anteverted.

frequency of the transducer, and/or bowel gas, may also be limiting factors.

Changes in endometrium

The endometrium is recognised from its position between the myometrium and the uterine cavity. Its appearance changes throughout

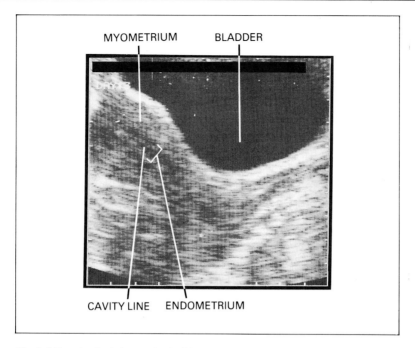

Fig. 2.4 Longitudinal view on day 3 of the menstrual cycle. The cavity line is clearly seen but the endometrium is thin and therefore hardly distinguishable from the underlying myometrium.

the menstrual cycle. Early in the cycle it is typically a thin area that is echo poor compared to the underlying myometrium (Fig. 2.4). As follicular activity increases, oestrogen levels rise and the endometrium consequently thickens and becomes more echo dense but is still less bright than the myometrial echoes (Fig. 2.5). Following ovulation, secretory endometrium is typically more echogenic than the myometrium (Fig. 2.6). However, these changes are highly variable, both between women and between cycles, and ovulation cannot be assessed accurately by studying ultrasonic endometrial changes.

If menstruation is delayed for any reason, the endometrium may be thickened such that it may be impossible to distinguish it from the decidual reaction which is seen with ectopic gestations (see Ch. 4).

Measurement of endometrial thickness

The endometrium tends to be qualitatively assessed rather than quantitatively. Although measurements can easily be made and may be of use in aiding subfertility management there are no thickness charts in general use. However, an endometrium that is more than 10 mm thick following ovulation suggests an adequate response.

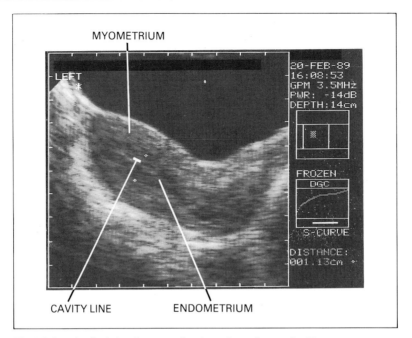

Fig. 2.5 Longitudinal view demonstrating the endometrium on day 10.

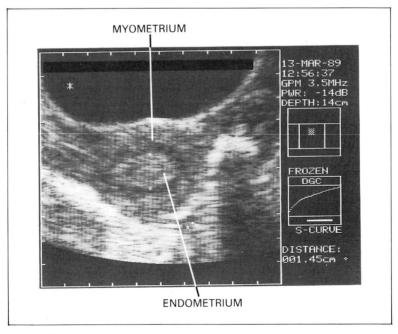

Fig. 2.6 Transverse view of the uterus on day 16 demonstrating a thickened, bright endometrium.

Measurements are most easily made in cross-section at the level of maximum endometrial thickness (see Fig. 2.6). The transvaginal route allows the endometrium to be visualised in greater detail and therefore enables measurements to be taken more accurately. Remember that the endometrial thickness measurement represents both anterior and posterior endometrial layers.

Fibroids

Fibroid is the common name for leiomyoma, a benign smooth muscle tumour of the uterus. Fibroids are very common, being present in over 20% of women over the age of 35 years. They are usually multiple (only 2% are solitary). They are most prevalent in the nulliparous and in dark skinned races. They are usually readily diagnosed clinically. Fibroids that are next to the cavity of the uterus (submucous) are difficult to visualise when scanned using the abdominal route but are readily diagnosed transvaginally. Such fibroids may prevent implantation or may cause recurrent miscarriages. Fibroids within the substance of the uterine muscle (intramural) or under the outer covering of the uterus (subserous) are easily detected abdominally. Transvaginally, fibroids which are large and/or calcified can be more difficult to assess as the

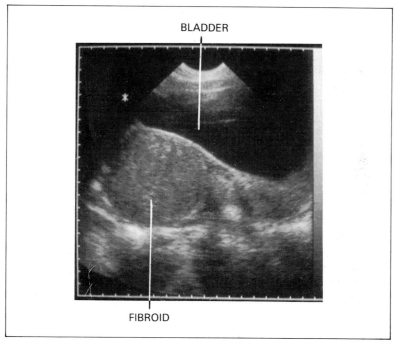

Fig. 2.7 Longitudinal view of the uterus demonstrating a fundal fibroid with a large fibrous component.

limited field of view can make visualisation and measurement difficult. Areas of calcification within the fibroid affect the transmission of the higher frequency sound beam of the transvaginal probe, degrading the images.

Ultrasonically fibroids usually appear as rounded, distinct masses of increased, decreased or similar echogenicity to that of the surrounding myometrium. This variability is due to the ratio of fibrous tissue (bright) to smooth muscle (dark) within them (Figs 2.7 & 2.8). They may indent the bladder if they are present on the anterior wall of the uterus. About 25% of fibroids become calcified and ultrasonically this is recognised by areas of high level echoes within the fibroid which may produce strong acoustic shadowing. A fibroid may be rimmed with calcification giving a strongly echogenic outline with an echo poor centre (Fig. 2.9). This may result in such a mass mimicking an ovarian cyst.

An echo poor posterior fibroid may also be confused with an ovarian cyst lying in the pouch of Douglas (Fig. 2.10). Always ensure that the presumed fibroid arises from the uterus and that it is separate from the ovaries.

Fibroids may grow so rapidly that they outstrip their blood supply producing central degeneration. In pregnancy, there is then bleeding

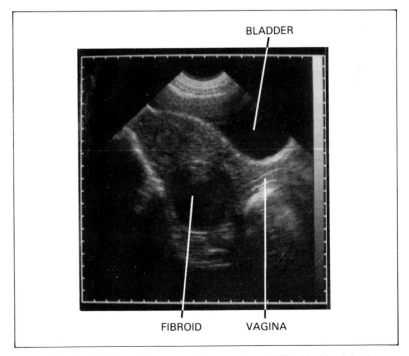

Fig. 2.8 Longitudinal view of the uterus with a posterior wall fibroid with minimal fibrous tissue.

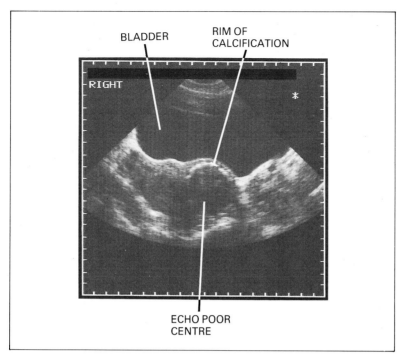

Fig. 2.9 Transverse view of the uterus with a left lateral fibroid demonstrating a rim of calcification.

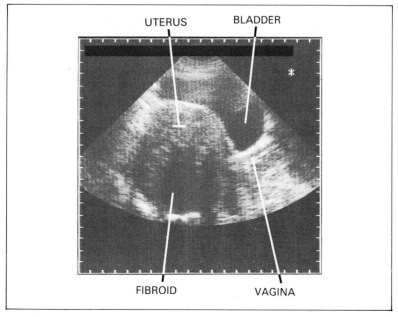

Fig. 2.10 Longitudinal view of the uterus with a posterior wall fibroid mimicking an ovarian cyst in the pouch of Douglas.

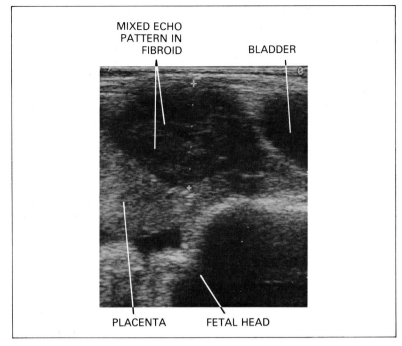

MIXED ECHO
PATTERN IN
FIBROID   BLADDER

PLACENTA   FETAL HEAD

Fig. 2.11 Longitudinal section of a pregnant uterus at 36 weeks gestation demonstrating red degeneration in a fibroid. The women was tender over the exact site of the fibroid.

into the centre of the fibroid (red degeneration) which can be acutely painful and difficult to distinguish clinically from an abruption. Ultrasonically, red degeneration is easily diagnosed (Fig. 2.11). If the woman is not pregnant, central degeneration is usually painless and results in an echo free area within the fibroid; this is known as hyaline degeneration.

After the menopause fibroids usually decrease in size. Serial measurements (six-monthly) may be requested as any increase in size may suggest malignant degeneration (leiomyosarcoma). This is very rare (0.2%) and apart from this size increase there are no characteristic ultrasound findings.

Indications for scanning fibroids are:

1. To confirm that a clinically detected pelvic mass is not an ovarian neoplasm.

2. To monitor the size of the fibroid, especially after the menopause.

3. In pregnancy

a. To detect cervical fibroids. Although only 3% of fibroids are cervical in position these will obstruct labour. The woman may present with an unengaged head in late pregnancy and will usually have been sent for a scan to exclude placenta praevia. If a cervical fibroid is discovered on a routine examination a further scan at 37 weeks will help the clinician to decide if the fetal head is below the level of the fibroid.

b. To aid in the differential diagnosis of abdominal pain. Red degeneration of a fibroid may mimic a placental abruption. The ultrasound appearances of red degeneration are usually obvious (Fig. 2.11) and it may be possible to demonstrate that the placenta is situated away from the site of the pain. If there is still doubt, anteriorly placed fibroids may be digitally palpated under ultrasound guidance and this will reproduce the woman's pain if it originates from the fibroid.

Intrauterine contraceptive devices (IUCDs)

The most common devices fitted are the Copper T and Copper 7; the Lippes loop is no longer manufactured but there are a few women who still wear them. Each device has a characteristic appearance.

Abdominal method

The uterine cavity is located in longitudinal section as described above. In this plane, both the Copper T and Copper 7 produce a continuous bright linear echo (Fig. 2.12), with a smaller bright echo superiorly,

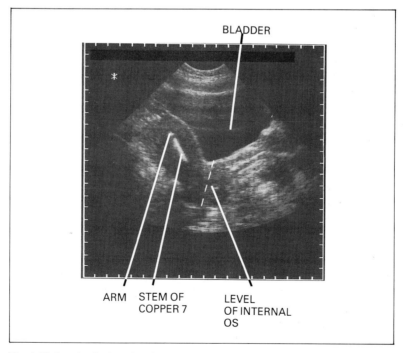

Fig. 2.12 Longitudinal section of the uterus demonstrating a Copper 7 intrauterine contraceptive device correctly positioned.

representing the T or the arm of the coil seen in cross-section. These echoes are considerably brighter than those obtained from the cavity line. With a cross-sectional view of the uterus the arm of the coil should lie at the fundus. The Copper T can be distinguished from the Copper 7 by visualising the point at which the arm of the coil joins the shaft: with the Copper T this is central and with the Copper 7 it is at one end. The Lippes loop will produce a series of very bright echoes (Fig. 2.13) representing the loops of the coil seen in cross-section.

The entire device should lie within the uterine cavity and within the body of the uterus — none should lie below the level of the internal os. Examination should ensure that the coil is correctly aligned and does not penetrate the myometrium. Copper 7 and Copper T IUCDs may rotate, so that the stem instead of the arm lies transversely within the uterus. If the IUCD is not seen within the uterus a careful search should be made of the pelvis but, once outside the uterus, IUCDs are often difficult to locate with ultrasound. In such situations an X-ray is indicated.

Women fitted with IUCDs have a high incidence of ectopic gestation should they become pregnant. If these women present with a missed period or irregular vaginal bleeding, then evidence of ectopic gestation should be carefully sought (see Ch. 4).

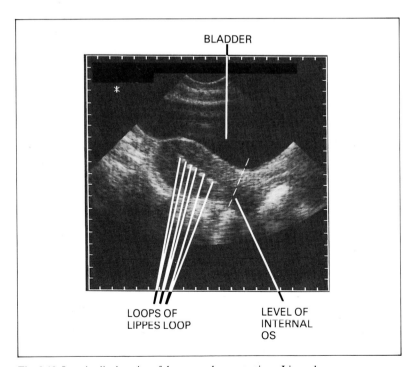

Fig. 2.13 Longitudinal section of the uterus demonstrating a Lippes loop.

Transvaginal method

The coil appears as described above. If the coil cannot be readily found, ensure the uterine cavity has been thoroughly examined across its full lateral extent. The transvaginal field of view is small relative to the abdominal field of view and therefore more sagittal slices are required to perform a proper examination.

Measurements of the uterus

Uterine measurements are best obtained abdominally, as the full length of the uterus can generally be visualised in one image. With the transvaginal probe the field of view is much smaller. In practical terms this means it is impossible to visualise the whole uterus in longitudinal section (and often cross-section), making accurate measurement impossible. However, uterine measurements are rarely of clinical importance.

The dimensions of the uterus increase with parity but decrease following the menopause. Measurements are taken in three planes. The longitudinal measurement (L) is made from the fundus to the level of the internal os. The transverse diameter (T) is obtained from a cross-section of the uterus at the widest part of the uterine body. The anteroposterior measurement (AP) is taken at the widest part of the uterus either in longitudinal or transverse section as this diameter is common to both planes (see Fig. 2.14). Typical uterine measurements are given in Table 2.1.

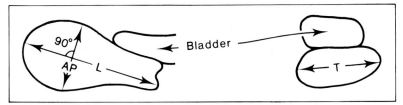

Fig. 2.14 Diagram demonstrating how to measure the uterus. Note that the AP measurement is obtained from the longitudinal scan.

Table 2.1 Normal uterine measurements (mm)

	Nulliparous	Multiparous	Postmenopausal
Longitudinal	<80	<95	<65
Anteroposterior	<40	<55	<18
Transverse	<40	<55	<18

(< = less than)

SCANNING THE OVARIES

The most difficult problem in ovarian or follicular scanning, from the operator's point of view, is actually locating the ovaries. Once this has been achieved, the rest is comparatively easy.

The ovary usually lies posterolateral to the uterus, anterior to the internal iliac artery, vein and ureter and medial to the ovarian vessels (Fig. 2.15). Ultrasonically, the vessels and the ureter provide the most useful landmarks. The internal iliac artery pulsates, and this easily distinguishes it from the ureter which lies immediately anterior to it. The ureter is visualised as a tubular structure with an echo free lumen. Very small, bright echoes can often be seen moving through the ureter. This sparkling is due to the peristaltic passage of urine. The ovarian vessels are also pulsatile and form a sheath of fine black lines that enter the ovary laterally (Fig. 2.16).

Abdominal method

The ovaries are most easily found by scanning the pelvis in planes at right angles to the long axis of the uterus. Use a probe with a small head

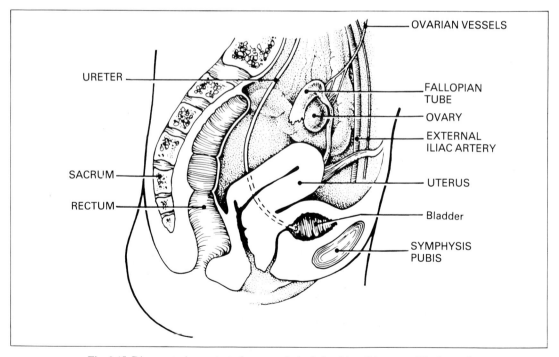

Fig. 2.15 Diagram to demonstrate the anatomical relationships of the ovary. The internal iliac artery cannot be visualised on this section because it is at right angles to the plane of the paper.

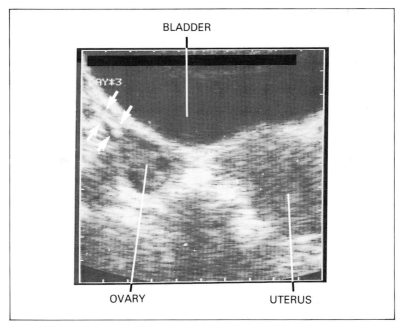

Fig. 2.16 Transverse view of the pelvis demonstrating the ovarian vessels entering the left ovary. Note the small follicles seen on day 3.

such as a sector, phased array, annular array or small convex curvilinear. Place the probe in the midline of the pelvis to obtain a longitudinal section with the bladder on the right of the screen. Locate the long axis of the uterus as described above. Rotate the probe through 90° such that a cross-sectional view of the uterus is obtained. By sliding the probe towards the fundus the ovaries are visualised lateral to the uterus as oval structures that are less echogenic and less homogeneous in echo pattern than the uterus (Fig. 2.17). To confirm that these structures are ovaries the ovarian vessels must be visualised entering laterally (Fig. 2.16). Having obtained a cross-sectional view, the longitudinal view is now easily obtained by rotating the probe slowly through 90° whilst keeping the ovary in view. The ovary should now be visualised lying anterior to the ureter and the internal iliac artery.

Unfortunately the ovaries do not always lie in this standard position. One or both may lie in the pouch of Douglas, or above the level of the uterine fundus when they often lie just below the skin surface. If one or both are not obvious using the above method then you must use the blood vessels to lead you to the ovary rather than vice versa. Remember that the ovarian position must be constant in both planes. If you locate an ovary in transverse section in the pouch of Douglas it must also be in the pouch of Douglas in longitudinal section and not at the fundus.

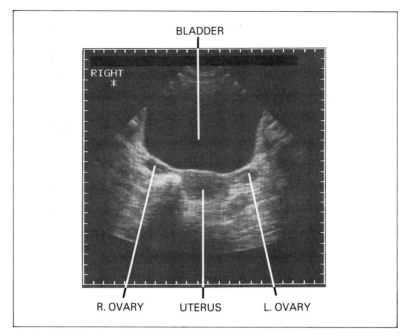

Fig. 2.17 Transverse view of the pelvis demonstrating the uterus and both ovaries.

Bowel gas may well obscure an ovary, especially if the latter is lying above the uterine fundus. Fluid-filled bowel can closely resemble an ovary (Fig. 2.18). Do not cheat if this is all you can find. If all else fails, check the woman has not had an oophorectomy!

Problems

Most problems are due to an inadequately filled bladder or an absent uterus. If the woman has had a hysterectomy, locating the ovaries may be difficult as the uterus is no longer present to provide a landmark and to displace the bowel superiorly out of the pelvis. Bowel gas is often a particular problem when the uterus is absent. Tipping the woman's head down may help. When the uterus is absent the obturator internus muscles are often mistaken for the ovaries (Fig. 2.19), but this will not occur if the ovarian blood vessels are identified. If the ovaries are not easily visualised follow the internal iliac vessels into the pelvis. The lower limit at which the ovaries may be found is marked by the levator ani muscle at its attachment to the vaginal vault (Fig. 2.20).

In postmenopausal women the ovaries are reduced in size and may be almost linear in shape (Fig. 2.21). Do not attempt ovarian scanning in the hysterectomised postmenopausal woman until you are confident of your abilities!

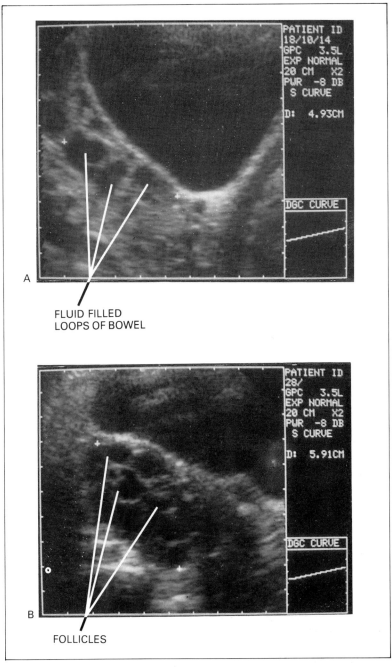

Fig. 2.18 (a) Fluid-filled loops of bowel mimicking the appearance of the multifollicular ovary seen in (b).

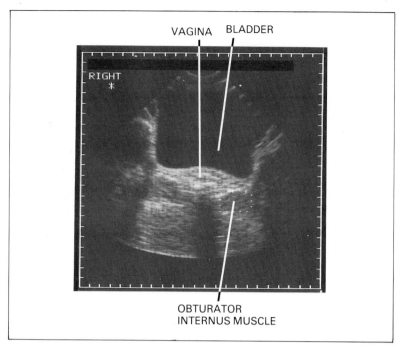

Fig. 2.19 Transverse section of the pelvis illustrating how the obturator internus muscle may be mistaken for the ovary.

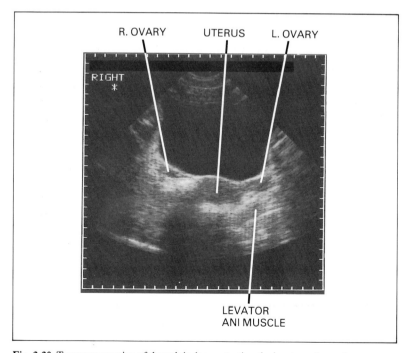

Fig. 2.20 Transverse section of the pelvis demonstrating the levator ani muscle.

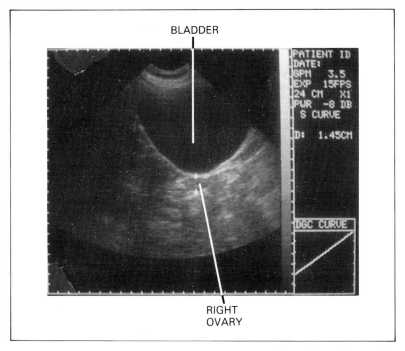

Fig. 2.21 Longitudinal section of an atrophic, postmenopausal ovary from a 62-year-old woman.

Transvaginal method

The fact that the ovaries do not occupy a standardised position in the pelvis, together with the small field of view available with the transvaginal probe, may make locating the ovaries difficult. Obtain a sagittal view of the uterus as described above, then pan the transducer laterally and rotate it slightly to obtain a parasagittal or oblique section of the pelvis.

Remember that, because the field of view is so small, it may be necessary to gently slide the transducer further up or down the vagina to visualise the ovary. If the ovary is not obvious then pan out toward the pelvic side wall until the ovarian blood vessels can be seen and then follow them to the ovary. The ovary is much easier to visualise when it contains follicles, as they are echo free.

Ovarian measurement

When examining the ovaries it is good practice to take measurements and calculate ovarian volumes. This trains you to define the end points of the ovary in each plane and also to look at the ovary more closely on each examination. Familiarity with the variants of the normal ovary will make detection of a possible abnormality more likely.

Ovarian size is generally expressed as a volume and this is calculated using the formula for the volume of the sphere:

$Volume$ (ml) $= \frac{4}{3}\pi r^3$

In practical terms it is much easier to use diameter measurements than radius measurements, so the above formula becomes:

$Volume$ (ml) $= length$ (cm) $\times width$ (cm) $\times depth$ (cm) $\times 0.5233$

The normal range of volumes is dependent upon the presence or absence of follicles in the premenopausal woman, but in the postmenopausal woman each ovary should have a volume of less than 10 ml. Furthermore, the ovaries should be approximately the same size, the volume of one being no more than twice that of the other. If such a discrepancy is found, make sure each ovary has been identified properly and that each diameter has been measured correctly. Remember that it is as easy to underestimate as to overestimate a diameter. If this happens, the appropriately measured ovary will appear abnormally large because the contralateral ovary was incorrectly measured. If there is still a significant difference in volume then even if the ovaries appear morphologically normal these women should be investigated further, usually by means of a laparoscopy. In addition to measuring ovarian volume, the ovaries should be carefully inspected. Any cystic structure is abnormal in a postmenopausal ovary, even if the woman is on hormone replacement therapy.

Ovarian volumes in the woman who is still ovulating will vary depending on the stage of the menstrual cycle at which she is examined. Early in the follicular phase the volumes should be comparable. There will obviously be a significant difference in volume between the ovary containing the leading follicle and the contralateral ovary in the days leading up to ovulation. Volumes in the luteal phase will depend on the size of the corpus luteum.

Women taking the combined oral contraceptive pill still produce follicles although these rarely exceed 8 mm in diameter. Larger echo free areas are usually simple cysts and, if less than 5 cm in diameter, all that is required is to rescan the woman in 6 weeks, i.e. at a different stage of her menstrual cycle. Women who are on the progesterone-only pill usually ovulate normally; the pill prevents implantation of the early pregnancy.

Measurement of ovarian volume is mainly used to screen women for ovarian cancer. The incidence of ovarian cancer increases with age, rising from 15/100 000 women below the age of 40 years to 50/100 000 women by the age of 70 years. Screening is generally offered to women over the age of 45 years. Detected early, ovarian cancer is curable but, as the ovaries lie deep within the pelvis, ovarian cancer usually presents at an advanced stage. Ovarian enlargement and/or unusual ultrasound appearances in one or both ovaries should suggest that further investigations are necessary to exclude a malignancy.

Ovarian masses

At the present time there are no ultrasonic findings that allow the certain distinction between benign and malignant tumours. Finding a thin-walled unilateral cyst, without solid areas and less than 5 cm in diameter, suggests benign disease (Fig. 2.22)—usually a follicular or a corpus luteal cyst (simple cysts). Re-examination in 6 weeks time, i.e. at a different phase of the menstrual cycle, will usually demonstrate that the mass is smaller or has disappeared.

Malignancy is suggested by the following:

- Thick-walled cysts
- Thick septa, particularly if they are incomplete
- Bilaterality
- Solid areas within the mass
- Excrescences, i.e. solid areas that appear to arise inside a cyst and then pass through its wall
- Ascites.

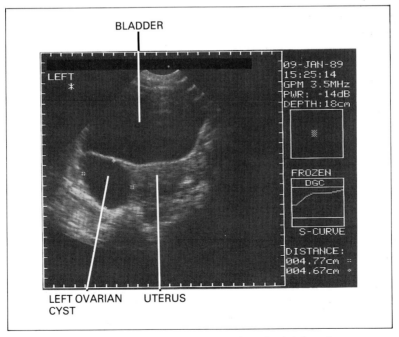

Fig. 2.22 Transverse section of the pelvis demonstrating a simple left ovarian cyst, measuring 4.8 cm by 4.7 cm.

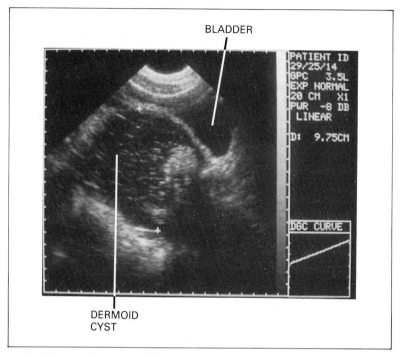

BLADDER

DERMOID
CYST

Fig. 2.23 Longitudinal section of the right ovary demonstrating a dermoid cyst. Note the complex pattern of echoes.

All of these changes, however, may be seen with benign tumours. Further problems arise in that blood clot or pus within the tumour may mimic solid areas. Dermoid tumours of the ovary (Fig. 2.23) are usually benign when discovered in premenopausal women. On ultrasound their appearances are very varied; they may be indistinguishable from simple cysts but more typically have a complex pattern of echoes due to their heterogeneous content. Dermoids may contain teeth, which give high level echoes, and sebaceous material and hair which cause bright echoes with marked attenuation of the sound beam such that the full extent of the tumour may not be appreciated. The pattern may mimic gas-containing bowel, but bowel usually demonstrates peristalsis. If ultrasound fails to confirm a clinically palpable mass the possibility of a dermoid should be considered and a plain X-ray ordered.

Our practice is to give descriptive reports and only rarely do we comment on the likely nature of the mass. Diagnosis and management of ovarian malignancy is beyond the scope of this book and of the majority of sonographers. What is important is the ability to differentiate between normal and potentially abnormal findings and alert the gynaecologist.

Ovarian masses in pregnancy

Ovarian cysts are very common in early pregnancy and are usually follicular or corpus luteal cysts. Whenever a cyst is found its size and appearance should be recorded. Providing the mass appears entirely cystic it is reasonable to rescan after 16 weeks gestation, after which time most cysts will have disappeared or will obviously be getting smaller. Cysts that are unchanged by 18–20 weeks gestation are usually surgically removed, as torsion or bleeding into the cyst is likely to occur in pregnancy.

Monitoring follicular development

About a third of infertile women fail to conceive because they do not ovulate. Ovulation can be monitored by using a temperature chart to look for a rise in early morning temperature, by biochemical means or by monitoring follicular development with ultrasound. The temperature chart method is often inaccurate. Biochemical means may involve the woman in daily collection of urine, blood or sputum. Commercially available home ovulation predictor kits are gaining in popularity but are often not sensitive enough for women with ovulatory problems. Ultrasound is quick, highly accurate and provides immediate results.

Predicting the time of ovulation is important for:

a. Timing of intercourse
b. Timing for artificial insemination, either by donor (AID) or husband (AIH)
c. Deciding the appropriate timing for oocyte retrieval for in vitro fertilisation (IVF) or gamete intra-Fallopian transfer (GIFT).

Method

The ovaries can be examined using either the abdominal or the transvaginal method. Wherever possible the transvaginal method should be used for follicular monitoring as the images obtained are far superior to those from abdominal examinations. This increases the accuracy of measurements of follicular diameter and allows much more detail of the primordial follicle to be seen.

Follicles appear as echo free areas within the substance of the ovary and can be visualised when they are 2 mm or more in diameter. Early in the menstrual cycle there will normally be several small follicles on one or both ovaries (Fig. 2.16). One follicle usually dominates and grows rapidly whilst the remainder become atretic. About 6 days before ovulation occurs the leading follicle will measure 6–10 mm in diameter (Fig. 2.24). Growth is then at a rate of about 2 mm per day until ovulation occurs at an average diameter of 22 mm (range 18–30 mm).

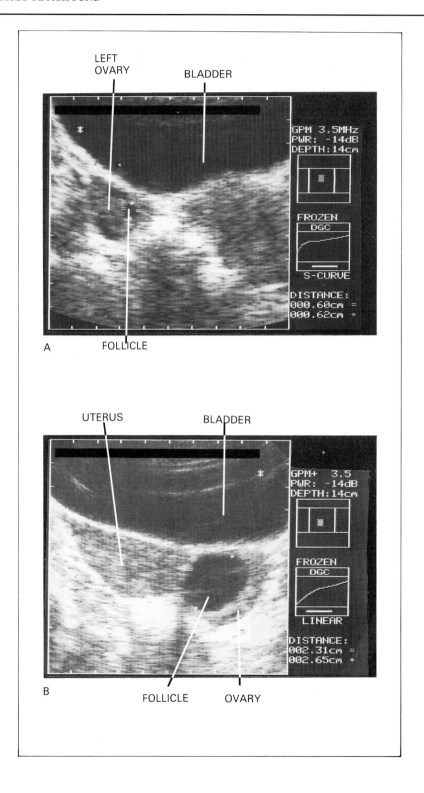

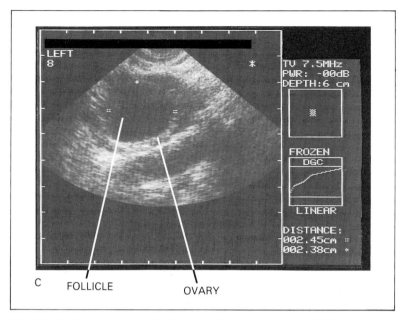

Fig. 2.24 (a) Transverse view of the left ovary demonstrating a 6 mm follicle on day 8. (b) Transverse section of the ovary demonstrating a 25 mm follicle on day 14. (c) The same ovary and follicle viewed transvaginally.

Ovulation is diagnosed by the collapse of the leading follicle(s). This may result in the complete disappearance of the follicle, or the resulting corpus luteum may be visualised at the site of the ruptured follicle (Fig. 2.25). The corpus luteum is a smaller structure than the follicle, often with rather irregular borders and containing internal echoes.

How and when to measure the follicle

Each ovary is visualised as described above and any follicular activity noted. The mean follicular diameter is the measurement used in reporting follicular size, and any follicles greater than 8–10 mm mean diameter should be measured at each examination. Having scanned the ovary, obtain the section that contains the maximum longitudinal diameter of the follicle. Measure this and then take another measurement at right angles to it on the same image. Rotate the transducer through 90° to obtain the maximum transverse diameter of the follicle. Measure this and then take another measurement at right angles to it on the same image. Calculate the average of these four measurements to obtain the mean follicular diameter. Follicles are not always spherical in shape, especially when the bladder is very full or the follicle is compressed against the pelvic wall. These factors are compensated for by measuring the follicular diameter in four planes.

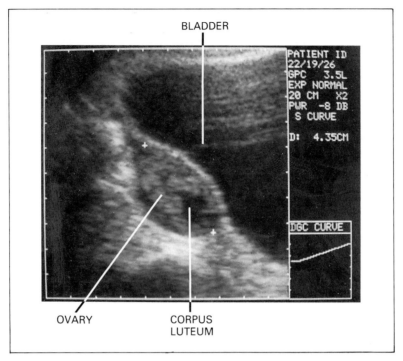

Fig. 2.25 Longitudinal section of the ovary demonstrating the corpus luteum. Note the irregular border.

Serial measurements are best plotted on appropriately designed charts that allow easy and quick interpretation (Fig. 2.26).

In women with regular, 28-day cycles the first scan should be performed 8 or 9 days after the first day of the last menstrual period (LMP). At this stage, a follicle of about 8–10 mm should be expected. Scanning on alternate days should then continue until ovulation has occurred. It is, of course, necessary to continue scanning until the follicle disappears or until the corpus luteum can be seen, rather than assume that this will occur when a follicle of 22 mm has been reached. This is important, as not all follicles of more than 18 mm in diameter will actually rupture. These follicles trap the mature ovum and prevent its release into the Fallopian tube — the luteinised unruptured follicle (LUF) syndrome. Ultrasonically, these follicles stay approximately the same size or regress slowly. The LUF syndrome may be the cause of infertility in women who are apparently ovulating by biochemical means. The LUF syndrome can only be diagnosed by ultrasound or operative means.

In women with irregular cycles it is still necessary to start scanning on day 8. In the absence of a follicle of 8 mm or more it is reasonable to

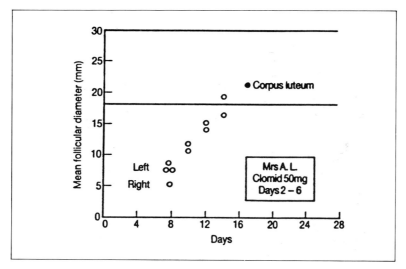

Fig. 2.26 A chart to aid ovulation induction. The small follicle seen in the right ovary on day 6 and two of the follicles in the left ovary become atretic. Ovulation occurs between days 14 and 16.

defer the repeat scan for 4 days. Once a follicle of 10 mm or more is visualised then scanning should be on alternative days as above.

Anovulation is diagnosed when:

- No follicles are observed throughout the cycle
- Growing follicles do not reach 18 mm mean diameter during the cycle
- Follicles of more than 18 mm mean diameter persist throughout the menstrual cycle. Follicles that achieve 18 mm or more in diameter and do not collapse are usually examples of the luteinised unruptured follicle (LUF) syndrome. These follicular cysts may persist into the next cycle and will delay or prevent ovulation. A scan on day 2, prior to commencing ovulation induction therapy, may be requested in these patients to ensure that the cyst has gone.

Stimulated cycles

Ovulation may be induced by a variety of drugs, the most commonly used being clomiphene (Clomid) or gonadotrophins (Pergonal or Metrodin). Follicular development is dose dependent, the aim of management being to produce one or two mature follicles per cycle. Multiple mature follicles suggest too high a dose has been given. In gonadotrophin cycles ovulation will not occur spontaneously, but must be initiated by an injection of human chorionic gonadotrophin (HCG). This mimics the luteinising hormone (LH) surge in spontaneous cycles and causes ovulation.

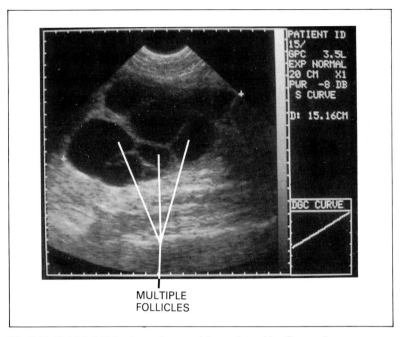

Fig. 2.27 Multiple follicles due to therapy with gonadotrophins (Pergonal).

HCG is usually administered when the leading follicle(s) has reached 18–20 mm. However, if there are more than three follicles of this size the administration of HCG is usually withheld as this may result not only in high multiple pregnancy but also in the hyperstimulation syndrome. This syndrome describes the development of multiple ovarian cysts, which may result in bleeding into the cysts, ascites and kidney failure.

In methods of assisted conception, however, it is desirable to harvest multiple ova, and the drug regimes are aimed to produce multiple mature follicles (Fig. 2.27). As the success rate of each stage of the in vitro fertilisation programme is low, multiple follicles are desirable to enable one or two embryos to be eventually replaced. Once the leading follicle(s) has reached 16–18 mm, HCG is given and the follicles are aspirated 36 hours later. In this situation hyperstimulation does not appear to occur as long as all the follicles are emptied.

Problems

The main problems encountered when monitoring follicular development arise because the ovary has not been thoroughly examined; follicles are therefore missed or incorrectly measured. It is important to take follicular diameter measurements as accurately as possible in order to assess whether follicular growth is appropriate or not. Ideally, the same operator should perform all the examinations, by the same route, during a cycle.

When many follicles are present it is important that they are all measured and that the relevant measurements taken in the longitudinal plane correspond to those of the same follicle in the cross-sectional plane. This requires a careful technique but can be achieved with perseverance.

It can sometimes be difficult to distinguish between a regressing follicle in a poor cycle and a corpus luteum in an ovulatory cycle, especially when more than 2 days have elapsed between examinations. A corpus luteum is generally smaller than a mature follicle and has a rather irregular internal border. Often, internal echoes will be visualised, representing blood clot within it.

CHAPTER THREE
Early pregnancy

Demonstration of a gestation sac within the uterus is the earliest
ultrasonic confirmation of an intrauterine pregnancy. Thickening of the
endometrium may be recognised prior to this but cannot be taken as
diagnostic of pregnancy. This appearance can be seen in the following
situations:

- The late luteal phase of the menstrual cycle
- In a very early intrauterine pregnancy, i.e. before the gestation sac
  can be resolved
- As a decidual reaction in association with ectopic pregnancy.

In addition, thickening of the endometrium can be confused with
retained products of conception within the uterine cavity.

The best images in early pregnancy are achieved by use of a
transvaginal probe. The higher frequencies used (6–7.5 MHz) improve
the resolution and allow early pregnancy features to be detected about
one week earlier than by the abdominal route. There is no evidence that
gentle transvaginal scanning is at all harmful, but the woman or her
doctor may wish you to carry out an abdominal scan in certain
situations. This should be performed using a probe with a small area of
contact (see Ch. 2).

THE GESTATION SAC

The gestation sac is the chorionic cavity of the developing pregnancy
and is visualised as a circular transonic area surrounded by a thick
bright ring. The sac usually lies at the uterine fundus and is
eccentrically placed. The ring and the eccentric position of the gestation
sac are best appreciated in a cross-section of the uterus. They are
important markers for confirming an intrauterine pregnancy.

The gestation sac may be visualised from about the time of the

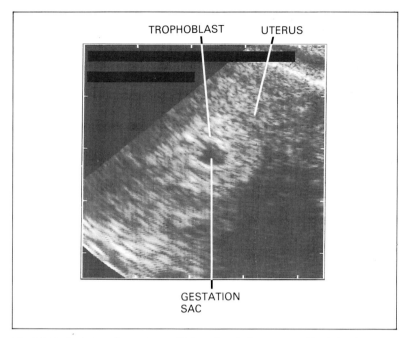

TROPHOBLAST   UTERUS

GESTATION
SAC

Fig. 3.1 Sagittal view of gestation sac 30 days after the last menstrual/period, using a transvaginal probe. Note the bright trophoblastic ring.

missed period using the transvaginal method (Fig. 3.1) and about a week later, i.e. 5 weeks amenorrhoea (Fig. 3.2), using the abdominal route. The advantages of using the transvaginal method are manifest with obese patients or those in whom the uterus is retroverted. The deterioration of the images caused by subcutaneous fat is avoided in transvaginal scanning.

Abdominal method

The bladder must be sufficiently full to cover the uterine fundus when attempting to visualise and measure a gestation sac abdominally. Locate the longitudinal axis of the uterus as described in Chapter 2. The gestation sac should be visualised towards the uterine fundus (Fig. 3.3). By sliding the probe and/or rotating slightly to either side, the maximum longitudinal axis (L) of the sac will be obtained. Rotate the transducer. If the sac has now disappeared, slide the probe either up or down the abdomen until you find it again, and obtain the section demonstrating the maximum transverse diameter (T) of the sac. Measure this from the frozen image. The maximum anteroposterior diameter (AP) can be measured from either the longitudinal or transverse section, as it is common to both views (Fig. 3.4).

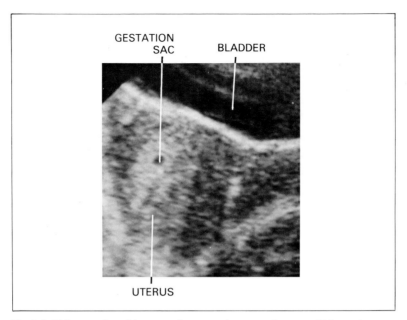

Fig. 3.2 Oblique section of the uterus demonstrating a gestation sac at 36 days using an abdominal sector scanner.

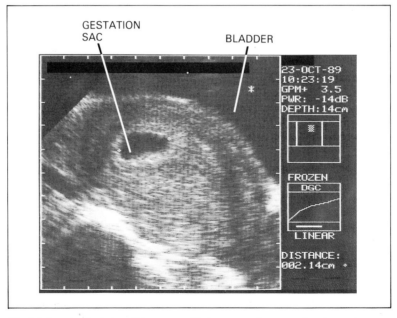

Fig. 3.3 Longitudinal view of the uterus with the cursors demonstrating the maximum longitudinal diameter of the gestation sac.

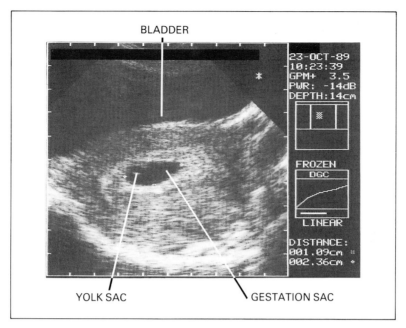

BLADDER

23-OCT-89
10:23:39
GPM+ 3.5
PWR: -14dB
DEPTH:14cm

FROZEN
DGC

LINEAR

DISTANCE:
001.09cm =
002.36cm +

YOLK SAC

GESTATION SAC

Fig. 3.4 Transverse section of the uterus from the same woman as Figure 3.3. The cursors now illustrate measurement of the maximum transverse and maximum anteroposterior diameters.

Transvaginal method

Obtain a true longitudinal (sagittal) view of the uterus as described in Chapter 2. If the gestation sac is not visualised, pan the transducer gently from side to side until the whole of the uterus has been examined and the maximum length of the gestation sac is displayed. Freeze the image and measure the maximum longitudinal diameter (L) together with the maximum anteroposterior diameter (AP) (Fig. 3.5a).

Rotate the transducer through 90° (keeping the gestation sac in view) in order to obtain a coronal section of the sac. It is important to appreciate that this is not equivalent to the transverse section obtained by means of the abdominal method (Fig. 2.3). Pan the probe across the width of the vagina until the gestation sac is visualised and then rock the handle of the probe until the maximum diameter of the sac is obtained in this plane. Freeze the image and measure the maximum transverse diameter (T) (Fig. 3.5b). It is good practice to also measure the longitudinal diameter, as this should correspond to that measured in the longitudinal (sagittal) section (Fig. 3.5a).

If the uterus is very anteflexed (or retroflexed) it may not be possible to rock the transducer sufficiently to obtain a true coronal section of the gestation sac. If this is not appreciated, measurements of the transverse diameter taken from this oblique view will be an overestimate. This is

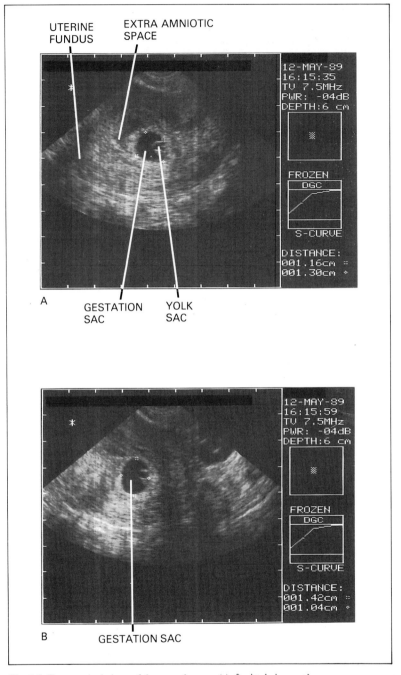

Fig. 3.5 Transvaginal views of the gestation sac. (a) Sagittal view — the cursors demonstrate measurement of the maximum longitudinal and anteroposterior diameters. (b) Coronal section — the cursors demonstrate measurement of the maximum transverse and longitudinal diameters. Note the extra-amniotic space seen above the gestation sac in (a).

important if it is necessary to estimate gestational age by means of gestation sac volume or if serial measurements of gestation sac volume are being used to determine if the pregnancy is ongoing. Apparent cessation of growth of the gestation sac over 1 week may be due to alteration of uterine position.

Calculation of gestation sac volume

The gestation sac volume may be calculated from the above measurements as follows:

Gestation sac volume (ml) = *L*(cm) × *T*(cm) × *AP*(cm) × *0.5233*

For the derivation of this formula, see Figure 3.6.

Figure 3.7 shows growth of the gestation sac. Gestation sac volume is used to estimate gestational age by reference to Table 3.1. Once the fetus can be identified within the gestation sac, a crown–rump length measurement should always be taken in preference as this is a more accurate means of estimating gestational age.

Uses of gestation sac measurements

- Confirmation of an intrauterine pregnancy
- Calculation of gestational age before the fetus is visible
- Diagnosis of an anembryonic pregnancy (see Ch. 4).

Viability

The pregnancy can only be said to be viable when fetal heart pulsations can be demonstrated within the gestation sac. These can be visualised vaginally from as early as 5 weeks post-menstrual age and abdominally from 6 weeks, i.e. 3 or 4 days before the fetus can be measured. Care

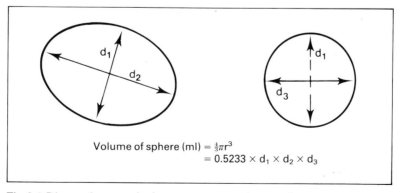

Volume of sphere (ml) $= \frac{4}{3}\pi r^3$
$= 0.5233 \times d_1 \times d_2 \times d_3$

Fig. 3.6 Diagram demonstrating how to measure gestation sac volume.

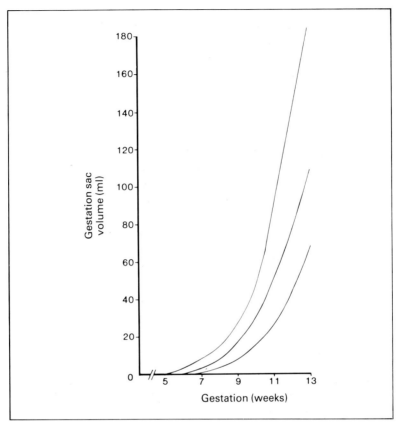

Fig. 3.7 Growth of the gestation sac with gestational age. (From Robinson RP (1975) British Journal of Obstetrics and Gynaecology 82:100, with kind permission of the author and publishers.)

Table 3.1 Growth of gestation sac volume

Amenorrhoea (days)	−2 sd	Mean (ml)	+2 sd
35–37	0.04	0.2	1.1
38–40	0.2	0.5	1.1
41–43	0.5	1.0	1.7
44–46	0.5	1.8	6.5
47–49	0.8	2.3	6.6
50–52	1.5	4.5	13.2
53–55	1.4	5.9	18.6
56–58	3.8	11.7	33.4
59–61	4.9	12.0	29.5
62–64	8.3	17.8	38.0
65–67	9.8	22.4	51.3
68–70	17.0	29.5	51.3
71–73	27.4	38.0	81.3
74–76	25.7	44.7	75.9

should be taken when confirming viability at this early stage as general background pulsations seen with many types of equipment can be falsely identified as pulsations from the fetal heart.

The absence of fetal heart pulsations within a fetal pole indicates fetal death and is therefore important in the diagnosis of missed abortion (see Ch. 4).

The embryo and fetus

Embryologically, the period from conception to the end of the ninth post-menstrual week is known as the embryonic period, whereas the remainder of pregnancy is termed the fetal period. In clinical medicine, however, the term 'fetus' is used throughout pregnancy.

The fetus can be visualised, and measured, from 40 days transvaginally. The most striking features at this stage are:

a. The 'blob' of the fetus (Fig. 3.8b)
b. The comparatively large yolk sac lying adjacent to the fetus (Fig. 3.9).

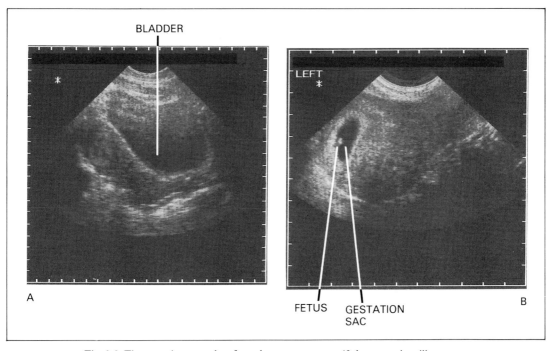

Fig. 3.8 These two images, taken from the same woman at 43 days gestation, illustrate the superior resolution of the transvaginal probe. In (a) it is difficult even to confirm an intrauterine pregnancy; with the transvaginal probe (b) the gestation sac and the fetus are clearly seen.

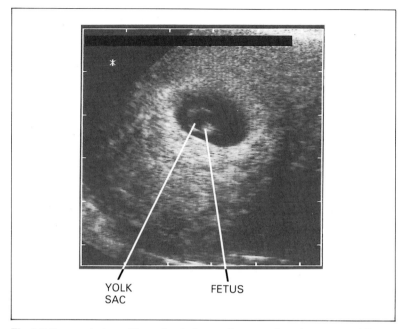

YOLK SAC   FETUS

Fig. 3.9 Transvaginal scan illustrating the large yolk sac seen in early pregnancy (40 days).

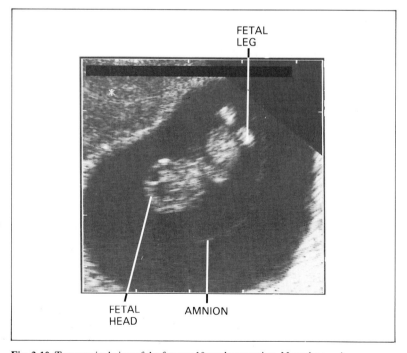

FETAL LEG

FETAL HEAD   AMNION

Fig. 3.10 Transvaginal view of the fetus at 10 weeks gestation. Note the amnion.

By 45 days the close proximity of yolk sac and embryo is lost because of the growth of the yolk stalk. The transformation of 'blob' to a recognisably human fetus is obvious, transvaginally, by about 10 postmenstrual weeks (Fig. 3.10).

The yolk sac

The yolk sac appears as a circular transonic mass within the gestation sac and can first be identified transvaginally at about 37 days. At this stage it is significantly larger than the embryo (Fig. 3.9). It is a prominent landmark to search for within the early gestation sac and because of its close association with the fetus it will automatically lead you to the fetus. The yolk sac floats freely in the chorionic cavity until the increasing size of the amniotic sac compresses it against the wall of the chorionic cavity. This occurs at around 11 weeks, making its identification difficult after this stage. Its diameter increases from 2 to 9 mm between 5 and 11 weeks. The yolk sac is of little practical significance ultrasonically. Care must be taken to ensure that it is not included in the measurement of the crown–rump length.

The amnion

The embryo lies within the amniotic cavity, which is bound by a membrane — the amnion. The amniotic cavity increases in size at a faster rate than the surrounding chorionic cavity. They do not achieve equal size until 14–16 weeks, when the amnion and chorion start to fuse. Sections of the amnion can often be identified ultrasonically as a fine line apparently floating within the gestation sac (Fig. 3.11) and may occasionally explain why amniotic fluid cannot be aspirated from a needle that is apparently within the gestation sac as it actually lies between the amnion and the chorion.

The placenta

Asymmetrical thickening of the decidual and trophoblastic layers surrounding the early gestation sac can be identified transvaginally from 6 weeks. This represents the developing placenta. By 8 weeks the placental site is easily identified (Fig. 3.12). Localising the placenta in the first trimester is necessary for chorion villus biopsy (see Ch. 9). Its position relative to the uterine cavity or the internal os is not predictive of the subsequent placental position.

Cystic areas within the uterine cavity can sometimes be identified (Fig. 3.13). These are thought to represent an implantation bleed, and the woman will usually have experienced some vaginal bleeding. They are very variable in size and occasionally appear alarmingly large, but, if the fetus is still alive, the size is not related to the pregnancy outcome.

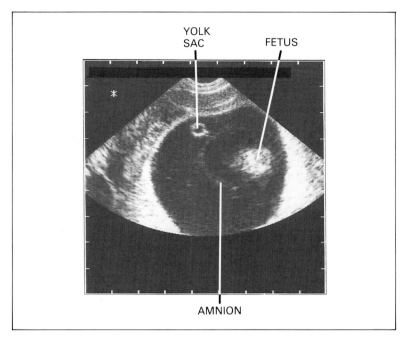

Fig. 3.11 Transvaginal scan demonstrating the amniotic membrane with the yolk sac lying between it and the uterus.

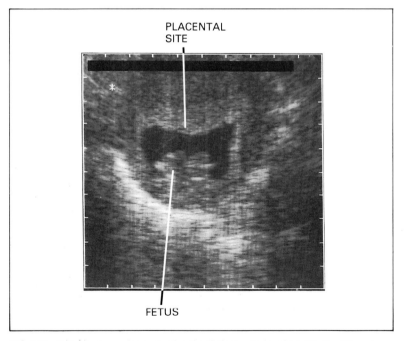

Fig. 3.12 Abdominal scan demonstrating the obvious anterior placental site at 8 weeks gestation.

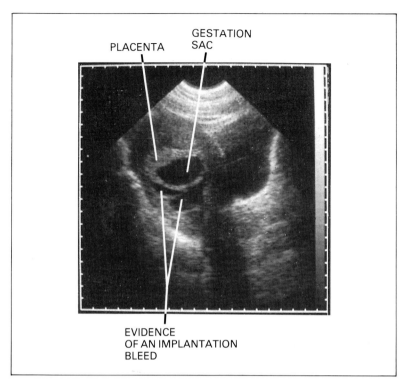

PLACENTA

GESTATION
SAC

EVIDENCE
OF AN IMPLANTATION
BLEED

Fig. 3.13 Longitudinal view of the uterus demonstrating evidence of an implantation bleed.

It is important to distinguish an implantation bleed from an empty second gestation sac (see 'Multiple gestation' below).

MEASUREMENT OF CROWN–RUMP LENGTH

Correctly performed measurements of crown–rump length are the most accurate means of estimating the gestational age. This is because the fetus grows very rapidly at this stage. However, accurate crown–rump measurements may be the most difficult measurements to obtain. The ability to correctly establish gestational age by this method depends solely on the operator obtaining a true, unflexed, longitudinal section of the fetus, with the end points of the crown and rump clearly defined. Appreciation of this only comes with experience, and for this reason we recommend that routine confirmation of gestational age should be performed in the second trimester (see Ch. 5).

Owing to fetal movement there can be no standardised technique for obtaining a crown–rump length. Firstly, find a longitudinal section of the uterus and gestation sac. Slide (if scanning abdominally) or pan (if

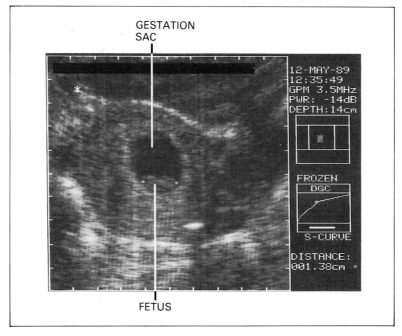

GESTATION
SAC

FETUS

Fig. 3.14 A view demonstrating the long axis of the fetus. The cursors demonstrate how to measure the CRL, which is 14 mm — equivalent to 7 weeks and 3 days.

scanning transvaginally) the probe slowly to each side until pulsations from the fetal heart can be seen. Slowly rotate the probe, keeping these pulsations in view, until the long axis of the fetus is obtained (Fig. 3.14). Once the fetal spine can be easily identified, i.e. from about 9 weeks, then this should be used as a guide in assessing true fetal length. The aim is to examine the fetus with the full length of its spine positioned directly anteriorly or posteriorly, thereby enabling you to assess any degree of flexion. Measurements are taken (from a frozen image) from the top of the head (crown) to the end of the trunk (rump) using the on-screen calipers (Fig. 3.15). The CRL measurement should be plotted on Figure 3.16. If the value lies within the normal range then the woman's menstrual dates are accepted. If the woman has no dates, or the value is outside the normal range, then the gestational age is established from the table in Appendix 4.

Problems

Abdominal method

Any degree of flexion of the fetal spine will produce an underestimate of the crown–rump length when linear calipers are used (Fig. 3.17). Should the fetal spine be lateral, the degree of flexion may be difficult to

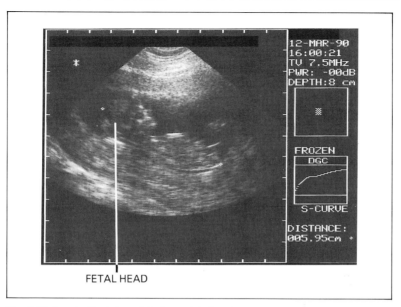

Fig. 3.15 Longitudinal view of the fetus with the spine posterior. The cursors demonstrate the measurement of the CRL, which is 60 mm — equivalent to 11 weeks and 6 days.

estimate. When scanning abdominally, alteration of the angle of the probe relative to the maternal abdomen may bring the spine into a more anterior, or posterior, position, thus making accurate measurement possible. When the fetus remains obstinately curled, you have four choices:

1. Sit and wait
2. Underestimate the crown–rump length by using the linear calipers along the flexed length (Fig. 3.17). This is not to be recommended under any circumstances
3. Measure the flexed length using on-screen non-linear measuring facilities often labelled 'length' (Fig. 3.18)
4. Use the linear calipers to measure the parts of the fetal length that are in straight sections, and then add them together (Fig. 3.19).

The accuracy of methods 3 and 4 will depend on your perception of the degree of flexion of the fetus. In theory, method 3 should be the most accurate. However, the caliper system is often very sensitive or obstinate (or both) and you will tend to overestimate the true measurement. Method 4 horrifies all purists (usually quite rightly) but is actually often a better, although less scientific, compromise.

When you have gained sufficient experience compare the three active alternatives on the same fetus. It is a salutary experience to discover

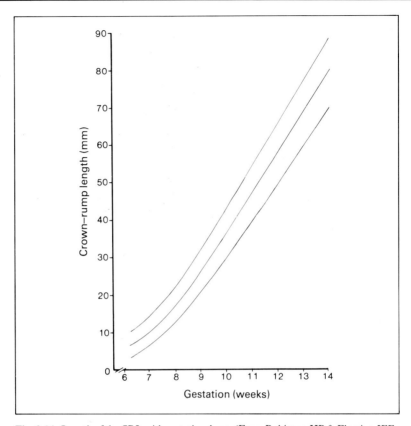

Fig. 3.16 Growth of the CRL with gestational age. (From Robinson HP & Fleming JEE (1975) British Journal of Obstetrics and Gynaecology 82:702, with kind permission of the authors and publishers.)

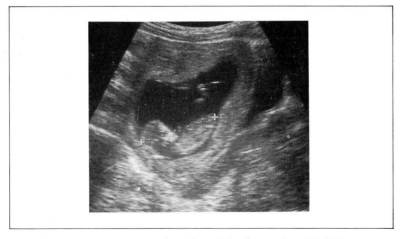

Fig. 3.17 Longitudinal section of a flexed fetus. Using linear calipers the CRL measures 56 mm which underestimates the true length by 14 mm (see Figs 3.18 & 3.19).

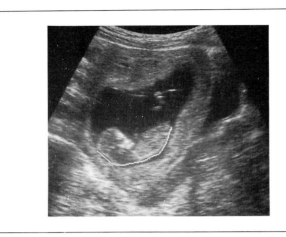

Fig. 3.18 This is the same image as Figure 3.17. Measurement of the CRL is made using non-linear calipers along the flexed length of the fetal spine giving a value of 70 mm.

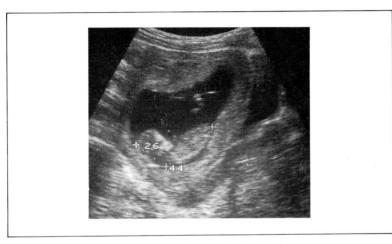

Fig. 3.19 This is also the same image as Figure 3.17. The CRL measurement is made by measuring the linear parts of the fetus separately (crown to shoulder, shoulder to rump) and adding the results together. The CRL of 70 mm is the same as that obtained from Figure 3.18.

how easy it is to produce errors of 10–15 mm simply by measuring incorrectly.

With increasing gestational age the fetus is more likely to be found in a flexed position. After 12 weeks postmenstrual age this generally makes assessment of the gestational age by crown–rump length inaccurate. Inaccuracies of 7–10 days can easily be obtained. We recommend that measurement is delayed until after 15 weeks, when the biparietal diameter can be easily and accurately obtained, rather than using crown–rump length measurements between 12 and 15 weeks.

Transvaginal method

The above problems of flexion are just as relevant using this method. The lack of manoeuvrability of the probe within the vagina is a major problem when the fetal spine is not optimally placed. You often cannot move the probe sufficiently to manipulate a lateral spine into an easier position for measurement. This is one of the most serious limitations of the transvaginal route.

MULTIPLE PREGNANCY

Multiple gestation sacs can be identified as early as singleton sacs, i.e. from 4 weeks transvaginally and from 5 weeks abdominally. However, the presence of a gestation sac does not indicate a viable pregnancy, but merely confirms an intrauterine pregnancy. It is therefore better to wait until two, or more, viable *fetuses* can be demonstrated before congratulating the parents. Unfortunately, not all viable twin pregnancies confirmed in the first trimester will go on to deliver twin infants, as the conception rate is about double that of the twin delivery rate. Approximately 30% of twin pregnancies that have been shown to be viable in the first trimester will lose one fetus. These points are important to remember when discussing early ultrasound findings with the parents.

Having diagnosed a twin pregnancy always make sure you have not missed an elusive triplet. The woman's confidence tends to falter if another fetus is discovered at every ultrasound examination. She will rarely return for a fourth appointment!

The incidence of congenital abnormalities is higher in monozygotic twins than in dizygotic twins or singleton pregnancies. The incidence of intrauterine growth retardation is also higher in multiple pregnancies than singleton pregnancies. For these two main reasons ongoing multiple gestations require careful ultrasound monitoring throughout pregnancy.

Problems

Not all cystic areas within the uterus are gestation sacs and it is important to distinguish between the following:

1. A genuine multiple gestation (Fig. 3.20).
2. Twin sacs due to artifact (Fig. 3.21). This artifact, which is known as a lateral artifact, is particularly likely to occur if a linear array

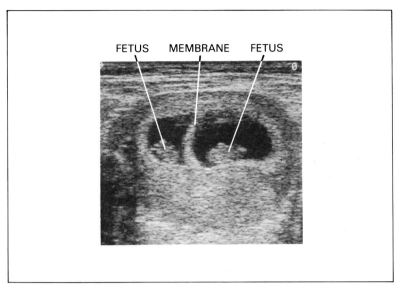

Fig. 3.20 Twin gestation sacs at 8 weeks amenorrhoea (abdominal transducer). Fetal heart beats were seen in both fetuses. The obvious dividing membrane probably means that the fetuses are dizygotic (non-identical).

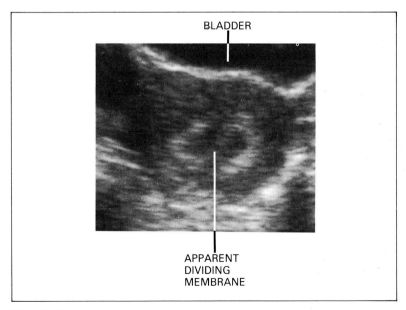

Fig. 3.21 Transverse view of the uterus obtained abdominally, demonstrating the lateral artifact that mimics twin gestation sacs.

probe is used in early pregnancy. It is readily recognised, as the two apparent sacs are only seen in transverse section.

3. An implantation bleed accompanying a singleton pregnancy (Fig. 3.13).

4. The extra-amniotic space. The gestation sac does not completely fill the cavity of the uterus until approximately 10 weeks gestation and therefore a space may be visualised between the sac and the cavity line (Fig. 3.5a). This space follows the contours of the cavity and does not have the echogenic ring characteristic of the gestational sac.

A kidney-shaped gestation sac will produce the appearance of twin sacs when viewed in certain sections. If this is a single sac then the two 'sacs' must join up at some point. Careful scanning of the sac(s) in several planes perpendicular to each other will determine if this is truly a multiple gestation.

A genuine twin gestation will usually demonstrate distinct and separate sacs. The sacs are generally adjacent but of differing shape and, if the fetuses can be visualised, they will generally lie in different planes and move independently. Rare exceptions are:

a. Monoamniotic twins — both fetuses lie within a single amniotic sac and there is no dividing membrane between them.

b. Conjoined twins — both individuals move together, being partially fused. These are also obviously monoamniotic.

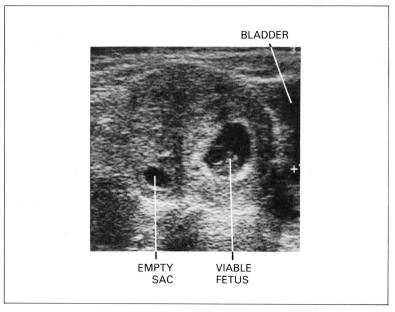

Fig. 3.22 A 7 week twin pregnancy. One sac contains a viable fetus and the other has a blighted ovum.

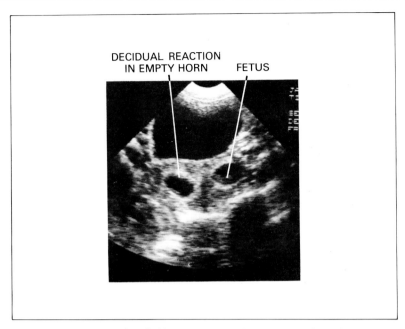

Fig. 3.23 Transverse section of a bicornuate uterus with a pregnancy in one horn.

Multiple sacs will not always contain viable fetuses. Identifying a viable singleton pregnancy together with an empty second sac is therefore common (Fig. 3.22), especially if there has been some vaginal bleeding. Reassurance to the woman as to the viability of the surviving fetus is obviously important but further explanation of the original twin conception must depend upon the individual situation.

BICORNUATE UTERUS

Figure 3.23 demonstrates a singleton pregnancy in a bicornuate uterus. The empty horn will exhibit a decidual reaction (Fig. 3.23) but may also show a collection of fluid within its cavity. The diagnosis of a bicornuate uterus is suggested by interrupted endometrial echoes on the transverse scan and by a transverse uterine diameter of more than 8 cm. Care must be taken to differentiate between (a) a bicornuate uterus with a singleton pregnancy and fluid within the cavity of the empty horn and (b) an early twin pregnancy in a normal uterus.

CHAPTER FOUR
Complications of early pregnancy

Apart from routine booking ultrasound examinations, the most common reasons for ultrasound in early pregnancy are vaginal bleeding and abdominal pain. Where ultrasound facilities are unavailable, the management of these women depends upon clinical examination and pregnancy testing.

Terminology

Abortion is the medical term for loss of pregnancy before 28 completed weeks of gestation. This includes both termination of pregnancy and spontaneous abortions. Miscarriage is a lay term for spontaneous abortion. However, as most women associate abortion with termination of pregnancy it is kinder to use the term miscarriage when dealing with women who may be losing a much wanted pregnancy.

Threatened abortion

Women who present with painless bleeding and a closed cervical os are diagnosed clinically as having a threatened abortion. The cause of the bleeding cannot be further resolved without the use of ultrasound, which will decide whether the pregnancy is ongoing or not.

Missed abortion and anembryonic pregnancy

A missed abortion is a pregnancy in which embryonic or early fetal death has occurred. It is unclear at present whether a pregnancy ever develops where no embryonic tissue forms at all within the blastocyst (a true anembryonic pregnancy), or whether the embryonic disc starts to develop but dies at a very early stage. For the sonographer this is a philosophical problem as such detail is beyond the current resolution of ultrasound. For practical purposes the terms anembryonic pregnancy

64

and blighted ovum are interchangeable and are used to describe a failed pregnancy in which no fetal pole can be found. This is in contrast to a missed abortion, in which the fetal pole is visible but no fetal heart beat is seen.

Over 60% of missed abortions and anembryonic pregnancies are associated with a chromosomal abnormality in the conceptus. Eventually these pregnancies will abort spontaneously although this may not occur until 12–13 weeks gestation.

Inevitable/incomplete abortion

Women who present with bleeding in the first trimester and in whom the cervical os is found to be open on vaginal examination have either lost or will lose their pregnancy.

If the pregnancy is still within the uterus but the cervical os is open this is termed an inevitable abortion, whereas if the conceptus has been partially expelled (usually recognised by the passage of clots) this is termed an incomplete abortion.

In both these groups of women the treatment is to remove the remaining products of conception under general anaesthetic. Ultrasound examination is therefore of no value in women in whom the cervical os is open in the first trimester, as these pregnancies are doomed and the management is decided purely on clinical grounds. However, ultrasound examinations are occasionally requested in order to help the women come to terms with the inevitability of their situation. Such women commonly have had either several miscarriages or have conceived as the results of fertility treatment.

Complete abortion

As the term suggests, the entire pregnancy has been expelled from the uterus. The history will be one of vaginal bleeding with the passage of clots, representing products of conception. The clinical findings are of a normal-sized uterus and a closed cervical os. Complete miscarriages probably only occur in women who are less than 6 weeks or more than 16 weeks pregnant. Ultrasound may be requested to firmly exclude products of conception.

Ultrasound appearances

Ultrasound examination will allow the differentiation between a live pregnancy and a missed abortion or anembryonic pregnancy, and is therefore an important aid to the management of threatened abortion. The fetus grows very rapidly, doubling its length each week of early life. This development is reflected in the varying ultrasound appearances found in the first trimester. You will not be able to diagnose pregnancy failure appropriately until you appreciate the ultrasound findings at a given gestation, with given equipment, in normal pregnancy.

The presence of a fetal pole together with fetal heart activity will confirm a viable pregnancy. With a transvaginal probe an intrauterine gestation sac can be identified from about 4 weeks gestation and a viable fetus from about 40 days (6 weeks) gestation. At this gestation the sac volume is about 0.5 ml. Using the abdominal route, a gestation sac can be seen from 5 weeks gestation and the fetal pole from 7 weeks gestation when the sac volume is about 3 ml. (See Table 3.1).

If the pregnancy is a missed abortion, no fetal heart activity will be detectable in the embryonic pole, and evacuation of retained products can be safely carried out. The ultrasonic appearances vary from a normal gestation sac and fetus without detectable fetal heart activity to a crumpled sac and fetus (Fig. 4.1). Incomplete abortions with retained products of conception do not show evidence of a gestation sac, but high level echoes arising from dead tissue are seen within the cavity (Fig. 4.2).

The only problem that arises is in trying to distinguish an anembryonic pregnancy from an early normal pregnancy. The woman's menstrual history cannot be relied upon because:

• The date of the last menstrual period may not be known

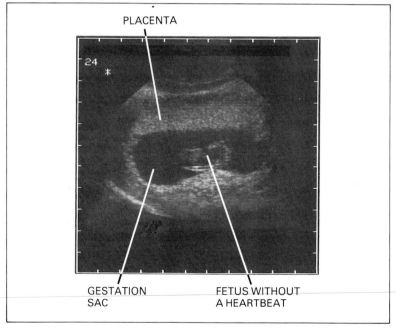

PLACENTA

24

GESTATION
SAC

FETUS WITHOUT
A HEARTBEAT

Fig. 4.1 Transvaginal scan performed at 8 weeks amenorrhoea, demonstrating a missed abortion. There was no fetal heart activity and the fetus is crumpled.

- She may have an irregular cycle
- She may have experienced bleeding in early pregnancy
- She may have recently stopped the oral contraceptive pill.

Even if none of these apply, up to 40% of women will demonstrate fetal measurements inappropriate for the postmenstrual age — this is taken to mean that conception has not occurred exactly 14 days after the last period (see Ch. 5).

The finding of an empty gestation sac on ultrasound therefore has to be resolved along the following lines. Measure the gestation sac volume as detailed in Chapter 3. The change in gestation sac volume relative to gestational age and crown–rump length is tabulated in Table 4.1 on page 68. If the gestation sac volume exceeds 3.0 ml a diagnosis of anembryonic pregnancy can be made with confidence either transvaginally or abdominally.

The fetus will only be visualised in pregnancies with gestation sac volumes of 1–3 ml with good equipment (usually a transvaginal probe) and an experienced operator. Therefore if the gestation sac volume is less than 3 ml we recommend that the woman should be rescanned in 1 week. At the repeat examination the sac volume should have doubled and the fetus should be seen and the heart beat demonstrated. In the case of an anembryonic pregnancy the sac will remain empty (Fig. 4.3).

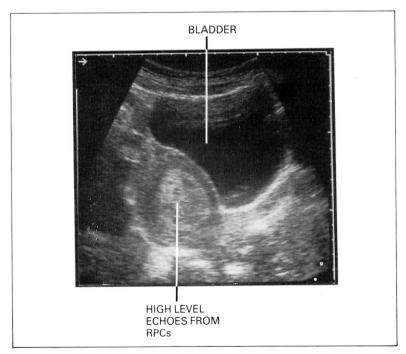

BLADDER

HIGH LEVEL
ECHOES FROM
RPCs

Fig. 4.2 Longitudinal view of a uterus containing retained products of conception (RPCs).

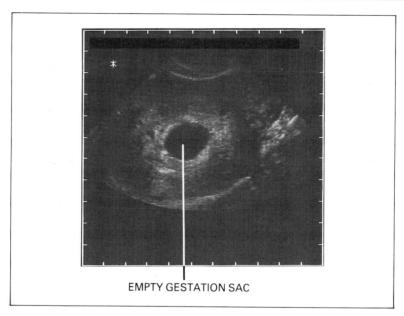

EMPTY GESTATION SAC

Fig. 4.3 Transvaginal scan demonstrating an empty gestation sac. The sac volume was 3.2 ml and no fetal parts were visualised.

Table 4.1 Gestational age related to GSV & CRL

Weeks. Days	GSV (ml)	CRL (mm)
5.0	0.2	
5.4	0.5	
6.0	1.0	
6.4	1.8	
7.0	3.0	10
7.4	5.2	14
8.0	7.5	17
8.4	10.2	19
9.0	17.5	25

Multiple conception

Multiple gestation sacs can be identified as early as singleton sacs. As twin pregnancies are subject to the same complications as singleton pregnancies it is possible to have a combination of a viable pregnancy with a missed abortion or an anembryonic pregnancy. In Caucasian women, twin gestation sacs are said to occur in 1 in 40 spontaneous pregnancies in the first trimester although the delivery rate is 1 in 80. Bleeding in the first trimester in these women will result in abortion of the entire pregnancy in 17% of cases whilst a further 33% will lose one sac. The incidence of twins varies with race, mainly due to variations in the dyzygotic twinning rate rather than the monozygotic. It is highest in West African women who have a twin delivery rate of 1 in 20.

ECTOPIC GESTATION

Ectopic gestation is a life-threatening condition in which the diagnosis may be difficult for the clinicians because of the varying modes of presentation. If a tubal pregnancy ruptures, the woman will rapidly become shocked and the diagnosis is usually then obvious. Most ectopic gestations, however, present in a more insidious manner. The patient may not have yet missed a period or there may be up to 12 weeks amenorrhoea. There may be little or no pain and minimal vaginal bleeding. The diagnosis is usually only raised by having a high index of clinical suspicion as there may be few clinical signs. This effectively means that all female patients of reproductive age who are having intercourse and who present with vaginal bleeding and lower abdominal pain, however mild, should be assumed to have an ectopic gestation until proved otherwise. The following groups of women are particularly at risk of an ectopic gestation:

- Women who conceive whilst wearing an IUCD
- Women who conceive whilst taking the progesterone-only pill
- Women who have had tubal surgery, including sterilisation operations
- Women who have a history of pelvic inflammatory disease
- Women in assisted conception programmes.

Modern pregnancy tests (assays of the β subunit of HCG) are now widely available and become positive at conception plus 10 days, i.e. 4 days before the first missed period. Women with a negative β-HCG pregnancy test are either not pregnant or the pregnancy is so early that it is not responsible for the woman's symptoms.

All women with a positive β-HCG pregnancy test and the clinical suspicion of an ectopic pregnancy should have an urgent ultrasound examination. The role of ultrasound depends upon the equipment available.

Abdominal method

If abdominal probes are all that are available, the main role of the ultrasound examination is to confirm or exclude an intrauterine pregnancy. Although an intrauterine pregnancy can co-exist with an ectopic gestation (heterotopic pregnancy), this is extremely rare in spontaneous conceptions (1 in 30 000 pregnancies). Women undergoing assisted conception are more likely to have a heterotopic pregnancy and this must be borne in mind when scanning them.

In the absence of an intrauterine pregnancy other signs of an ectopic gestation should be sought. An extrauterine gestation sac with a fetus will only be visualised in about 5% of cases (Fig. 4.4). An adnexal mass, especially if associated with free fluid in the pouch of Douglas

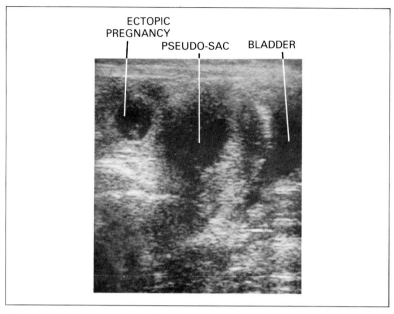

Fig. 4.4 Ectopic gestation with a viable fetus in an extrauterine site. The uterus contains a large pseudo-sac composed of decidual cast and blood clot.

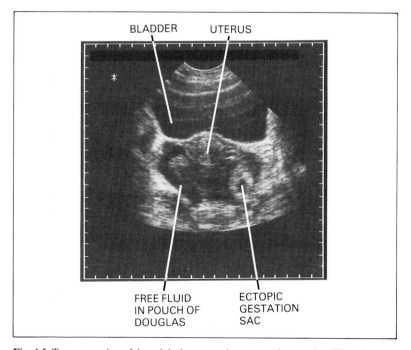

Fig. 4.5 Transverse view of the pelvis demonstrating an ectopic gestation. There is a visible extrauterine gestation sac and there is a large amount of free fluid (blood) in the pouch of Douglas.

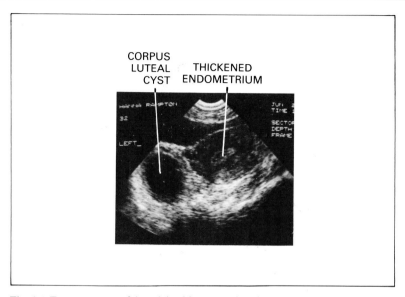

Fig. 4.6 Transverse scan of the pelvis with a corpus luteal cyst and thickened endometrium mimicking a decidual reaction.

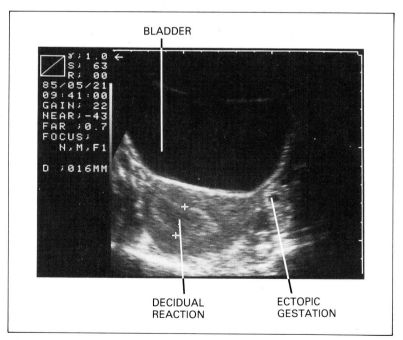

Fig. 4.7 Transverse scan of the pelvis. There is a right sided ectopic gestation and the uterus demonstrates an obvious decidual reaction.

(Fig. 4.5), is very suggestive of an ectopic pregnancy but this appearance can also be seen with a corpus luteal cyst (Fig. 4.6). Experienced operators may also be able to comment on the presence or absence of a decidual reaction (Fig. 4.7) but this appearance is unreliable as it may be mimicked by a thick endometrium seen in association with any cause of delayed menstruation.

Figure 4.4 illustrates the so-called pseudo-gestational sac. This is composed of a decidual cast and blood clot. If it is mistaken for a gestation sac then an ectopic pregnancy may be missed. Comparison with Figure 3.3 demonstrates that the true gestation sac has a thick bright rim surrounding it that is further thickened at the site of the future placenta.

Transvaginal method

Again, the exclusion of an ectopic gestation relies largely upon the demonstration of an intrauterine sac, which can be seen from about 4 weeks amenorrhoea by this means. The superior resolution of transvaginal probes allows more accurate assessment of the adnexae and the uterine cavity and hence many more ectopic gestations can be diagnosed or excluded. Figure 4.8 demonstrates an ectopic gestation containing a yolk sac diagnosed at 6 weeks amenorrhoea. A further

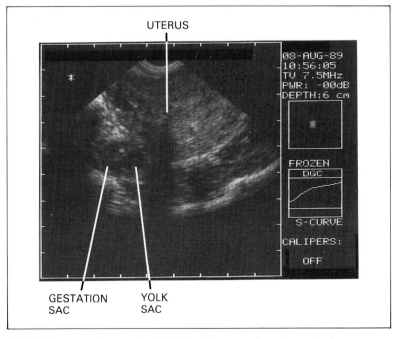

Fig. 4.8 Transvaginal scan performed at 6 weeks amenorrhoea, demonstrating an extrauterine gestation sac that contains a yolk sac.

advantage of the transvaginal method is that a full bladder is not required.

Widespread use of β-HCG pregnancy tests together with transvaginal probes should eliminate many of the unnecessary laparoscopies that had to be performed on early pregnancies that were below the resolution of abdominal ultrasound. An exciting development is the possibility of treating ectopic pregnancies by injections of methotrexate (which kills the trophoblast) under ultrasound control, thus avoiding surgery.

HYDATIDIFORM MOLE

The cause of this unusual tumour is unknown but it may be a neoplastic change in either an anembryonic pregnancy or a missed abortion. The woman usually presents to her doctor with painless vaginal bleeding. She may also have hyperemesis gravidarum (severe vomiting in pregnancy), a raised blood pressure and a uterine size that is larger than expected for her gestation. The main differential diagnosis is multiple pregnancy. Very rarely a twin gestation may present with one normal fetus and a mole. Moles are benign but they may become malignant (choriocarcinomata). Moles occur with a frequency of 1 in 3000 pregnancies in Caucasians but are more common in Asians (1 in 300 pregnancies).

The ultrasound diagnosis of a hydatidiform mole is usually easy. It has a classic 'snowstorm' appearance on B-mode scanning. On real time

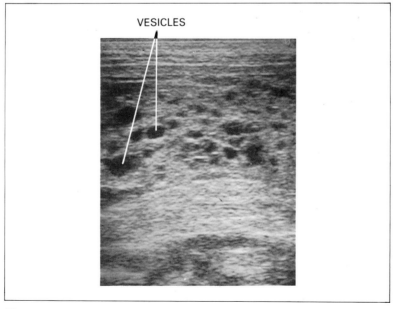

Fig. 4.9 Transverse section of a hydatidiform mole (abdominal scan).

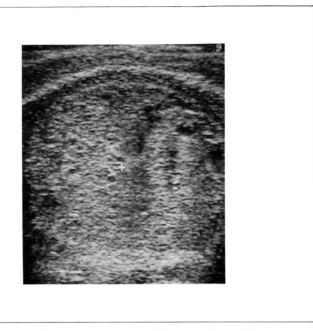

Fig. 4.10 Transverse section of a degenerating fibroid (abdominal scan). Note the similar appearance to Figure 4.9.

the small vesicles and the areas of haemorrhage are more obvious (Fig. 4.9). Although the diagnosis may be straightforward, the appearances of a missed abortion with hydropic degeneration (accumulation of fluid in the placenta) or of a degenerating fibroid may cause confusion (Fig. 4.10). Making the diagnosis of hydatidiform mole is important because after the mole has been evacuated from the uterus these women must have careful follow-up to exclude subsequent development of a choriocarcinoma. This is done by serial β-HCG estimations on blood or urine as these tumours are placental in origin and so produce β-HCG. β-HCG is only found in the blood or urine of women who are pregnant or who have trophoblastic disease (mole or choriocarcinoma). These women are usually advised not to become pregnant again for a year because earlier pregnancy increases the risk of the development of a choriocarcinoma. It is important that they should be scanned early in their next pregnancy to exclude a further mole.

THE INCOMPETENT CERVIX

An incompetent cervix is caused by the congenital absence of, or damage to, the circular layer of muscles that surround the internal os. It may result in miscarriage in the second trimester or preterm labour. It can be treated by insertion of a cervical cerclage at 12–14 weeks gestation, which will result in a term pregnancy in about 85% of cases. Unfortunately, insertion of the cerclage may cause a miscarriage. The diagnosis cannot be reliably made by any means, but recently serial ultrasound measurements of the internal os from 16 weeks gestation have proved to be of help.

Method

The internal os is best visualised by use of an abdominal transducer with a small head, with the bladder full. Obtain a longitudinal section of the uterus and then rotate the probe slightly until the cervical canal is visualised (Fig. 4.11). The length of the canal and the width of the internal os can be measured on a frozen image. Fortnightly serial measurements may then be made looking for a shortening of the canal or dilatation of the internal os.

Interpretation

The normal cervix should have a length of 2.5 cm or more from 10 weeks gestation until 36 weeks, and the width of the cervical canal at the level of the internal os should be less than 4 mm. Herniation of the

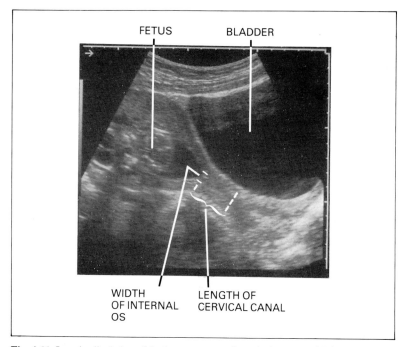

Fig. 4.11 Longitudinal view of the lower uterus and cervix demonstrating how to measure the width of the internal os and the length of the cervical canal.

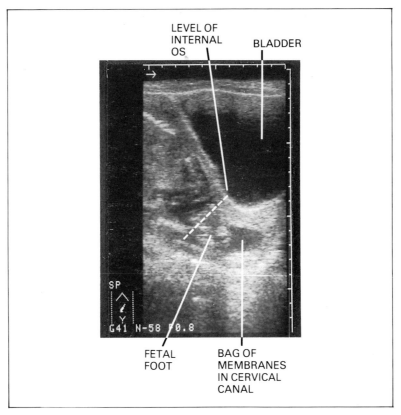

LEVEL OF
INTERNAL
OS

BLADDER

SP

G41 N-58 /0.8

FETAL
FOOT

BAG OF
MEMBRANES
IN CERVICAL
CANAL

Fig. 4.12 Longitudinal scan of the lower uterus and cervix demonstrating cervical incompetence. There is a bag of membranes prolapsed into the cervical canal and the fetus is attempting to block the internal os with its foot!

amniotic sac with or without fetal parts (Fig. 4.12) is associated with midtrimester miscarriage or preterm delivery in almost all women unless a cervical suture is inserted.

The finding of a cervix that is less than 2 cm in length or an internal os that is open to more than 8 mm in width predicts preterm delivery or midtrimester miscarriage in about 75% of cases. As yet, we do not know whether inserting a cervical cerclage into these women improves the outlook for the pregnancy.

CHAPTER FIVE
Estimation of gestational age

The most accurate way to calculate the length of pregnancy is by knowing the date of conception. Delivery would then be expected to occur 38 weeks (266 days) later. As most women are unaware of the date of conception, the first day of the last menstrual period (LMP) is used to calculate the expected date of delivery (EDD). This is done by applying Naegele's formula to the LMP as follows:

1. Add 7 to the days
2. Subtract 3 from the months
3. Add 1 to the years.

For example, if the LMP is 13.4.90 then the EDD is $(13+7).(4-3).(90+1)$, that is 20.1.91. This means that pregnancy is 40 weeks (280 days) long and assumes that conception occurs two weeks after the LMP.

The LMP is unreliable (and therefore Naegele's formula cannot be used) in the following circumstances:

- When the date of the LMP is not accurately known
- When the menstrual cycle is not 28 days long
- When the menstrual cycle is irregular
- When the woman has only stopped taking the combined oral contraceptive pill ('the pill') within the last 3 months
- When the woman has bled in early pregnancy.

This had led to the use of two terms:

1. Gestational age. This is the length of pregnancy based upon a reliable LMP, assuming that conception occurs 14 days later.
2. Postmenstrual age. This is the length of the pregnancy based upon the LMP, irrespective of its reliability.

THE USE OF ULTRASOUND

Several ultrasound parameters have been used to estimate gestational age. The most commonly used are:

- Gestation sac volume (see Ch. 3)
- Crown–rump length (see Ch. 3)
- Biparietal diameter
- Femur length
- Head circumference
- Abdominal circumference.

Use of these is as follows:

Gestational age (weeks)	Parameter
4–7*	Gestation sac volume
6–12*	Crown–rump length
12–15	Defer measurement
15–24	Biparietal diameter
	Femur (and circumference measurements)
24 weeks onwards	Gestational age cannot be accurately determined by ultrasound

* Recognition of a gestation sac from 4 weeks and a fetal pole from 6 weeks can only be achieved with a transvaginal probe (see Ch. 3).

All ultrasound examinations benefit from a methodical approach and this is especially true where measurements are required. However, an ultrasound examination should be more than a means of confirming gestational age as it provides an ideal opportunity for assessing fetal anatomy and therefore structural normality. Assessment of placental morphology, amniotic fluid volume and the interpretation of measurements may all be important pointers to potential problems in a pregnancy. We recommend the following sequence:

1. Determine the number of fetuses (see Ch. 3)
2. Determine the longitudinal lie of the fetus
3. Check the fetal heart is beating
4. Show the woman her baby's image on the screen
5. Take measurements of the fetal head
6. Return to a longitudinal section which demonstrates the full length of the fetal spine
7. Measure the fetal abdomen
8. Continue down the spine in transverse section to the sacrum. Find the femur and measure it.
9. Localise the placenta
10. Calculate gestational age and redate if necessary
11. Discuss the findings with the woman.

FINDING THE LONGITUDINAL AXIS OF THE FETUS

Place the transducer on the maternal abdomen to obtain a midline longitudinal section of the uterus. Slide the transducer to each side of the abdomen until the fetal head is visualised. Repeat the process to identify the fetal heart within the fetal chest. Slowly rotate the transducer, keeping the heart in view, until a longitudinal section of the fetal body is obtained. By sliding or altering the angle of the transducer with respect to the maternal skin a longitudinal section of the fetal spine will be obtained. Rotate the transducer such that the fetal head and body are visualised on the screen together as shown in Figure 5.1.

Knowing the relationship of the longitudinal axis of the fetus to the maternal abdomen establishes fetal lie and is an important preliminary to obtaining accurate measurements of the fetal head and abdomen.

THE BIPARIETAL DIAMETER (BPD)

The BPD is the most widely used ultrasound parameter in the estimation of gestational age. It is also the easiest to obtain, and on a routine basis is the most accurate. A single optimal measurement of the BPD will predict the gestational age to within ±5 days. It is more

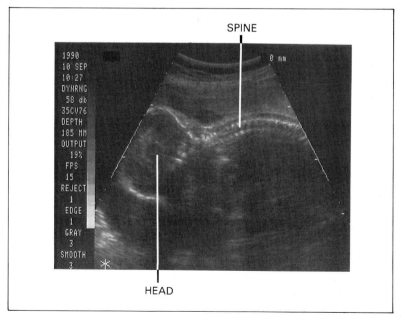

Fig. 5.1 Longitudinal section of fetal head and upper spine. This is the section required to determine the fetal lie.

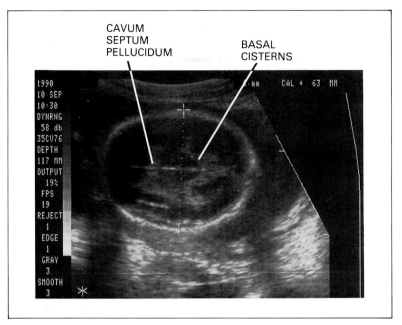

Fig. 5.2 Transverse section of the fetal head from which the BPD should be measured.

accurate at predicting the date of delivery than an optimal menstrual history. This last point justifies its use in all pregnancies.

The BPD is the maximum diameter of a transverse section of the fetal skull at the level of the parietal eminences. The correct section is demonstrated in Figure 5.2 and should include the following features:

- A short midline
- The cavum septum pellucidum
- The thalami
- The basal cisterns.

This level is recommended by the British Medical Ultrasound Society (BMUS) Ultrasonic Fetal Measurement Survey as the standard section from which to obtain a BPD measurement together with measurements of the head circumference (HC) and occipitofrontal diameter (OFD).

Measuring the BPD

Obtain a longitudinal section of the fetus as described above. By small sliding movements of the transducer on each side of the fetal spine a longitudinal section of the fetal head will be obtained which will demonstrate a strong midline echo (Fig. 5.3). By rotating the transducer through 90° a transverse section of the fetal head is obtained.

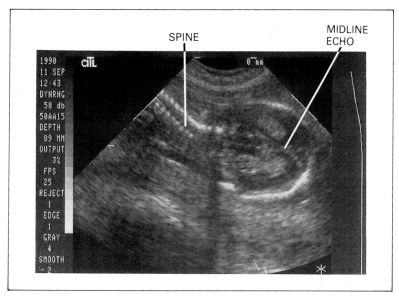

Fig. 5.3 A longitudinal section of the fetal head and spine demonstrating the midline echo. Rotating the transducer through 90° should produce the section demonstrated in Figure 5.2

If the midline is not in the exact middle of the section, angle the probe slightly. This corrects for the angle of asynclitism. Now assess the shape of the fetal skull and if it is not the required ovoid shape make minor rotational adjustments. If the features listed above are not evident when the midline and shape are correctly imaged, then the level of the section is wrong and should be corrected by small sliding movements of the probe.

The BPD is then measured on the frozen image. Place the horizontal component of the first on-screen caliper on the outer aspect of the proximal skull surface. Place the horizontal component of the second caliper on the inner aspect of the distal skull surface at right angles to the midline and at the widest diameter (Fig. 5.2).

Problems

1. BPD measurements in breech and transverse presentations

In the second half of pregnancy, BPD measurements obtained from fetuses presenting transversely or by the breech may be unreliable. In these presentations the fetal head may be dolichocephalic (long and narrow) in shape. This produces a BPD measurement which is artifactually small for gestational age. The head circumference measurement, however, is unaltered by presentation and is therefore reliable. Most ultrasonographers recognise the abnormal shape but if in doubt the cephalic index (see p. 92) should be measured. If it is less than 75, the BPD measurement should be ignored.

2. OP/OA position

Measurement of the BPD can only be obtained when the fetal head is in the occipito-transverse (OT) position, as the landmarks are best recognised when the midline echo is at 90° to the ultrasound beam. The BPD therefore cannot be measured if the fetal head is directly occipito-posterior (OP), directly occipito-anterior (OA) or deep in the maternal pelvis. Tilting the woman into a 45° head down position and/or filling the maternal bladder may displace and rotate the fetal head such that it can be measured. If this fails, estimation of gestational age may be made from measurement of femur length but we recommend rescanning the woman at a later date to ensure that the fetal head is normal.

3. Incorrect angle of asynclitism (Fig. 5.4b & e)

With real-time scanners the angle of asynclitism has to be guessed but this is easily done. If the angle is incorrect the midline echo does not lie centrally within the fetal skull. The angle of the probe to the maternal abdomen should be altered without sliding or rotating the probe.

4. Incorrect rotation (Fig. 5.4d & f)

This is readily recognised because the visualised shape of the fetal skull is not that of a rugby football—it is usually too round. Rotating the probe will correct the shape but you must be careful to maintain the angle of asynclitism.

5. Incorrect levels (Fig. 5.4a & c)

Sliding movements of the probe will alter the level of section. Be careful not to rotate or change the angle of the probe as you slide.

The recommendations from the British Medical Ultrasound Society are very recent. Previously, most workers used the section illustrated in Figure 5.4c. Measurement of the BPD should be exactly the same from the two sections although measurement of HC may be minimally different. The disadvantage of the recommended section is that it fails to demonstrate the cerebral ventricles. Cranial abnormalities will therefore be overlooked unless the operator specifically examines the cerebral ventricles after measuring the BPD.

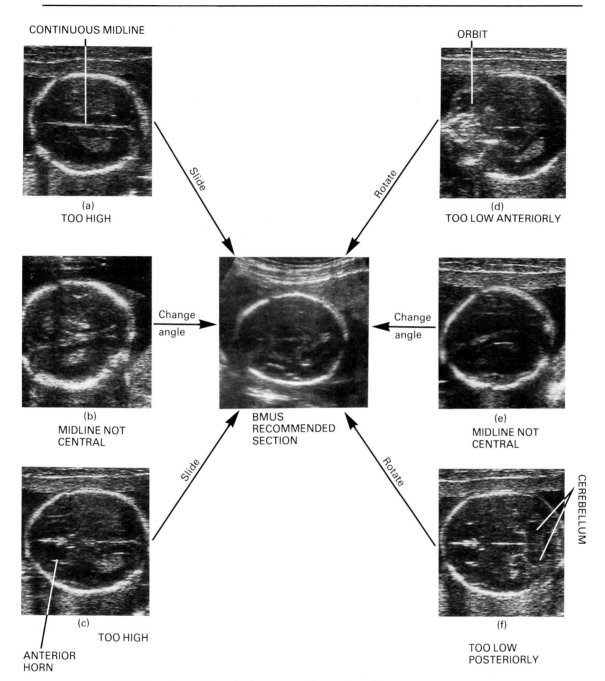

Fig. 5.4 Diagram illustrating how to move the transducer from various incorrect sections to obtain the correct section on which to measure the BPD.

Estimating gestational age from BPD measurements

BMUS Ultrasonic Fetal Measurement Survey recommended that all ultrasound machines should be calibrated at 1540 m/s and the biparietal diameter measured from outer to inner skull tables (Fig. 5.2). The reasons for this choice of outer to inner is explained in Chapter 15. You must be aware of the velocity at which your ultrasound machine calipers are set, and use appropriate charts. We do not rely upon estimates of gestational age produced by the equipment for the following reasons:

1. Estimation of gestational age should not be made from a single parameter.
2. Manufacturers do not always state the origin of the charts provided, and these may not be appropriate for the equipment.
3. Estimation of gestational age and monitoring growth require different charts (see below).

Figure 5.5 illustrates the change in the biparietal diameter with increasing gestational age. It was derived according to the recommendations given above. For statistical reasons it should be remembered that this chart should be used to determine if the measurement of the BPD is within the normal range for the postmenstrual age.

Estimation of gestational age should be made from charts in which the BPD is plotted on the x-axis (independent variable) and the gestational age is plotted on the y-axis (dependent variable), or from tables derived in the same manner (see Appendix 4). In practical terms this means that, having measured the BPD, you should plot it as on Figure 5.5. If it is outside the normal range for the postmenstrual age you should estimate the gestational age by use of the tables (Appendix 4).

MEASUREMENT OF HEAD CIRCUMFERENCE

Figure 5.2 illustrates the section required for measurement of the BPD. The HC is measured on the same section. Circumference is calculated by one of two basic methods:

1. *A method using a computer to sum the distances between a series of dots put around the perimeter of the fetal skull.* Using either a joystick, a roller ball or a light pen, the dots should outline the outer table of the skull. In some equipment a continuous trace is produced rather than a series of dots.
2. *The ellipse method.* Here, you place the first on-screen cursor on the outer table of the skull at the occiput. The second cursor is then placed on the outer table of the skull at the sinciput. Using the

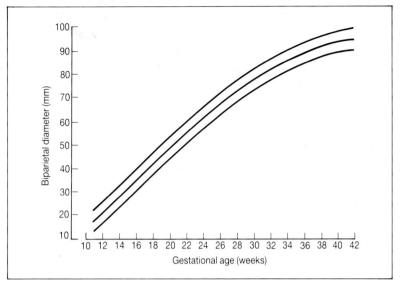

Fig. 5.5 Growth of the BPD (mean ± 2SDs) with increasing gestation. From Hadlock FP, Deter RI, Harrist RB Journal of Ultrasound Medicine 1: 97–104. This chart is reproduced full size in Appendix 5.

appropriate control, a ready formed ellipse of dots is moved out from between the two cursors until it matches the outline of the fetal skull (Fig. 5.6). On some machines adjustment of the site of the cursors can be made after the ellipse is formed to achieve a more exact match.

If your equipment does not have facilities for circumference measurements they can be calculated from measurement of the BPD and OFD. Figure 5.6 illustrates measurement of the OFD. The circumference is then calculated from the formula:

$$HC = 1.62\,(BPD + OFD)$$

The alternative to this is to use hard copy and a map measurer as described in Chapter 1.

Growth of the HC is illustrated in Figure 11.1 and Figure 2, Appendix 5.

MEASUREMENT OF ABDOMINAL CIRCUMFERENCE

Figure 5.7 illustrates the section on which the abdominal circumference is measured. The salient features are:

1. The outline is circular.
2. A short length of umbilical vein. This should be imaged so that it is centrally placed between the lateral abdominal walls and is a third of

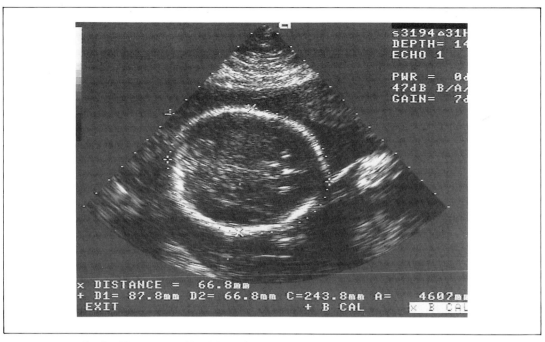

Fig. 5.6 Measurement of head circumference using the variable ellipse methods. The head circumference measures 243.8 mm. The OFD (+ . . . +) measures 87.8 mm. Note that the D2 distance (× . . . ×) of 66.8 mm does not represent the BPD as the lower cursor has been placed on the outer border of the skull table.

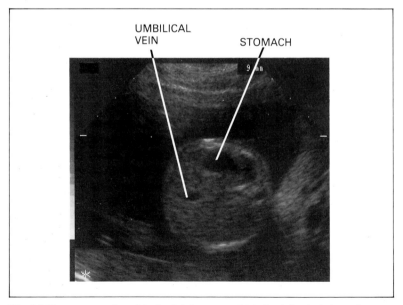

Fig. 5.7 Transverse section of the fetal abdomen on which the abdominal circumference should be measured.

the way along an imaginary line drawn from the anterior abdominal wall to the fetal spine.

3. The stomach is usually visualised as a transonic area in the left side of the abdomen.

Method

Obtain a longitudinal view of the fetus that demonstrates both the fetal heart and the fetal bladder. Slide the transducer laterally until the fetal aorta is visualised in its course through both the fetal chest and abdomen. Rotate the transducer through 90° at the level of the fetal stomach to obtain a cross-section. Ensure that the outline is circular by small rotational movements of the transducer. If the umbilical vein is not visualised as described above, make small sliding movements of the transducer to change the level of the section. Freeze the image.

The circumference of the abdomen is measured in the same way that the head circumference is measured.

If your equipment has only linear calipers then the circumference

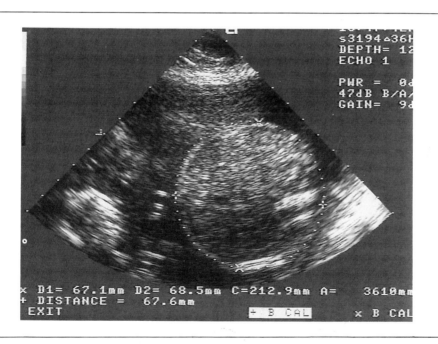

Fig. 5.8 Transverse section of the fetal abdomen demonstrating measurement of the APAD (+ . . . +) and TAD (× . . . ×). The circumference measurement derived from diameters is:

$$3.14 \, (\, 67.1/2 + 67.6/2 \,) = 211.5 \text{ mm}$$

which is very similar to the 212.9 mm derived from the variable ellipse method.

may be calculated from the transverse and anteroposterior diameters using the formula:

$$AC = 3.14 \, (TAD/2 + APAD/2)$$

Figure 5.8 illustrates the measurements of the TAD and APAD. Growth of the AC is illustrated in Figure 11.1, and Figure 3, Appendix 5.

Problems

1. Directly anterior fetal spine

When the fetal spine is directly anterior it may not be possible to visualise the fetal aorta in which case a long length of the fetal spine should be used to obtain a longitudinal view. In transverse section the umbilical vein will not be seen, as it lies in the acoustic shadow produced from the fetal spine (Fig. 5.9a). In early pregnancy it is nearly always possible to slide the transducer to a more lateral position on the maternal abdomen or to dip one end of the transducer to allow the umbilical vein to be imaged (Fig. 5.9b). Alternatively you can complete the remainder of the examination by which time the fetus may well have moved into a more favourable position.

In later pregnancy it is sometimes necessary to measure the AC with the spine directly anterior. In this situation the stomach has to be used as the sole landmark.

2. Non-circular outline

It is not infrequent to obtain the correct section for the AC but to have a fetal limb indent the outline. In this case, as long as the landmarks are correct and the outline would be a circle but for the indentation, the section can be used. In tracing the circumference the cursor must follow the indentation, otherwise a falsely low measurement will be obtained. With ellipse measuring systems this is not possible so you must wait until the fetus moves into a position that allows a circular outline.

Oval outlines indicate an oblique cross-section, which can be rectified by slight rotational movements of the transducer.

Fetal breathing movements can markedly alter the shape of the fetal abdomen, especially in late pregnancy. Fetal breathing movements are usually intermittent, and with patience a section can be obtained in fetal apnoea.

3. Late pregnancy

In late pregnancy it is often not possible to fit the entire outline on the screen. In this case the appropriate section should be obtained and

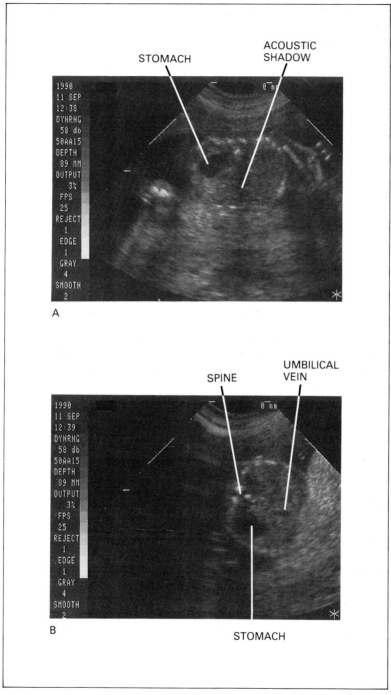

Fig. 5.9 (a) Transverse section of the fetal abdomen demonstrating how the acoustic shadow from an anterior fetal spine obscures the umbilical vein. (b) The same fetus imaged from a lateral aspect on the maternal abdomen.

displayed as centrally as possible with the minimum amount of outline
beyond the edges of the screen. As the section is circular the outline
may be measured. Some machines will not allow measurements beyond
the frozen real-time image, in which case a Polaroid picture must be
taken and the outline traced with a map measurer (see Ch. 1). It is
better not to report an AC than to use the underestimate that will be
obtained if an incomplete section is traced.

FEMUR LENGTH

This measurement is as accurate as the BPD in the prediction of
gestational age. It is useful in confirming the gestational age estimated
from BPD measurements and can often be obtained when fetal position
prevents measurement of the BPD. As examination of intracranial
anatomy is an important part of all ultrasound examinations,
measurement of femur length should not replace that of the BPD as the
sole predictor of gestational age. The femur can be measured from 12
weeks gestational age to term.

Method

Find a transverse section of the fetal abdomen and slide the transducer
caudally until the iliac bones are visualised. At this point a cross-section
of the femur is usually seen. By keeping this bright echo from the femur
in view, rotate the transducer until the full length of the femur is
obtained. To ensure that you have the full length and that your section
is not oblique, soft tissue should be visible beyond both ends of the
femur and the bone should not appear to merge with the skin of the
thigh at any point (Fig. 5.10).

The measurement of the femur is made from the centre of the
'U'-shape at each end of the bone. This represents the length of the
metaphysis. It is good practice to obtain measurements from three
separate images of the same femur. These should be within 1 mm of
each other.

Growth of the femur is illustrated in Figure 5.11, and Figure 4,
Appendix 5.

If the femur length is used to estimate gestational age, the measurement should be plotted on Fig. 5.11. If it lies outside the normal range
for the postmenstrual age or if the woman's dates are unreliable then
estimate the gestational age from the tables in Appendix 4.

Problems

The femur length is an easy and very accurate measurement to obtain if
the above simple guidelines are followed.

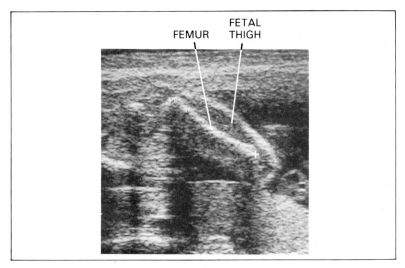

Fig. 5.10 The fetal femur. Note that soft tissue is visible beyond both ends of the bone. The femur length is the distance between the caliper markers.

The estimation of gestational age obtained from measurements of femur length should agree with that obtained from the measurement of the BPD. If the femur length is small compared to the BPD then all the long bones should be carefully measured to exclude dwarfism (see Ch. 8).

ROUTINE ESTIMATION OF GESTATIONAL AGE

At the time of the routine 16–20 week ultrasound examination we recommend that the minimum measurements that should be made are those of the BPD and the femur. There are four possibilities:

1. The measurements of the BPD and the femur fall within the normal limits for the postmenstrual age when plotted on appropriate charts. This confirms the postmenstrual age.

2. Both measurements fall outside the normal limits for postmenstrual age. In this case you estimate the gestational age from the BPD using the tables (see Appendix 4) and then re-plot the femur length for the estimated gestation. If it is within normal limits you should then determine the new EDD. In this case it is good practice to also measure the HC and AC for further confirmation.

3. The BPD falls within normal limits for the postmenstrual age but the femur length is below these limits. In this case you must measure the HC and AC and repeat the measurements of the BPD and femur. If all the measurements but that of the femur agree with the

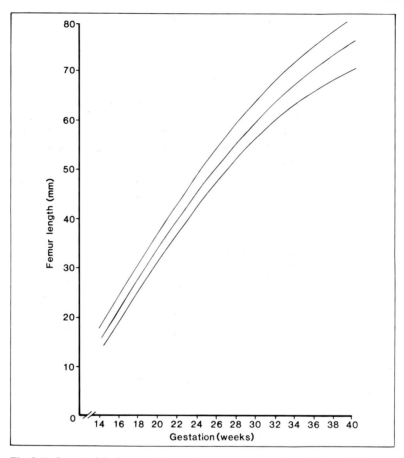

Fig. 5.11 Growth of the femur with increasing gestational age. From Warda A H, Deter R L, Rossavik I K 1985 Obstetrics and Gynaecology 66: 69–75. This chart is reproduced full size in Appendix 5.

postmenstrual age you should suspect a limb reduction deformity (see Ch. 8).

4. The femur falls within the normal limits for gestational age but the BPD is below such limits. Again you must repeat the measurements and also measure the HC and AC. If the HC and BPD are both below the normal limits you should look for spina bifida or microcephaly (see Ch. 7). If all the measurements are appropriate but for the BPD you should determine the cephalic index:

Cephalic index = BPD/OFD × 100 = 80 ± 5

An index of less than 75 is seen in cases of dolichocephaly (usually associated with a non-cephalic presentation) and makes the BPD measurement unreliable for estimating gestational age. The rare condition of craniosynostosis (see Ch. 7) should also be considered.

An index of more than 85 is seen in brachycephalic heads and also makes use of the BPD for estimating gestational age unreliable.

The cephalic index is constant throughout pregnancy.

When to estimate gestational age

We hope it is apparent from the above that we believe that all women should have their gestational age confirmed by ultrasound. Ultrasound estimation of the date of delivery is better than the estimation obtained from women with impeccable menstrual histories and this justifies the routine use of ultrasound.

The optimal time to perform the routine examination is 16–20 weeks gestation. Examination at this time has the following advantages:

- It gives an accurate prediction of the gestational age
- It allows the diagnosis of all multiple pregnancies
- Placental localisation at this time is reliable (see Ch. 10)
- Most major structural anomalies can be recognised at this time (see Chs 7 and 8). By following the sequence we suggest most major abnormalities should be excluded during a routine examination
- The optimal time to perform estimation of maternal serum AFP is 16–18 weeks. If the test is performed after ultrasound estimation of gestational age it reduces the number of false tests due to inaccurate dating or multiple pregnancy
- Demonstration of a viable healthy fetus increases maternal-fetal bonding.

Examination in early pregnancy may, of course, be necessary for complications of pregnancy (see Ch. 4) or to reassure the very anxious mother.

Determining gestational age in multiple pregnancy

If the fetuses are of different sizes then measurements from the larger fetus should be used to determine the gestational age.

WHAT TO DO WITH THE 'LATE BOOKERS'

Prediction of gestational age by ultrasound cannot be accurately made after 24 weeks gestation. Women who attend after this time fall into three categories:

1. Those in whom all measurements correspond with the postmenstrual age. These women do not need further ultrasound examinations unless clinically indicated.

2. Those who have an unreliable menstrual history or in whom fetal size is less than that predicted by menstrual dates. In these women an

accurate EDD cannot be predicted. They should have serial ultrasound examinations to monitor fetal growth. As long as growth continues it is usually unnecessary to interfere with the pregnancy because of fetal concern.

3. Those in whom fetal size is greater than that predicted from the menstrual history. These women should be rescanned three to four weeks later and the rate of growth studied. It is usually possible to predict an EDD after the second examination. Women with maternal diabetes mellitus may have large fetuses and pose a special problem if they book late (see Chs 11 and 12).

CHAPTER SIX
Normal fetal anatomy

The recognition of fetal anomalies by ultrasound is based upon a sound understanding of the appearances of normal fetal anatomy. Although it is possible to describe the techniques for demonstrating the various organs, by far the best way of learning the anatomy is to spend as much time as possible studying normal fetuses. In general, the earliest time at which the fetus can be studied for structural anomalies is 16–18 weeks, but when you are starting to study normal anatomy the organs in the 20–26 week fetus are easier to visualise.

Although it is necessary to examine the entire fetus and other uterine contents in detail it is often not feasible to do this in a set order. If a fetal organ presents itself it should be studied immediately as if examination is postponed the fetus may then be in an unfavourable position. A mental checklist is necessary to ensure that the study is complete. We should suggest that the measurements are carried out early in the examination so that they are not forgotten.

THE FETAL HEAD

Examination of the intracranial anatomy should follow on naturally after taking the measurements of the BPD and HC (Ch. 5). Demonstration of normal cerebral ventricles will exclude the most common cranial abnormalities.

The cerebral ventricles

Figure 6.1 is a schematic diagram that illustrates the ventricular system. Cerebrospinal fluid (CSF) is produced by the choroid plexus and circulates through the ventricular system, around the brain and around the spine. It is absorbed by special areas of the arachnoid. Excess production or failure of absorption leads to communicating

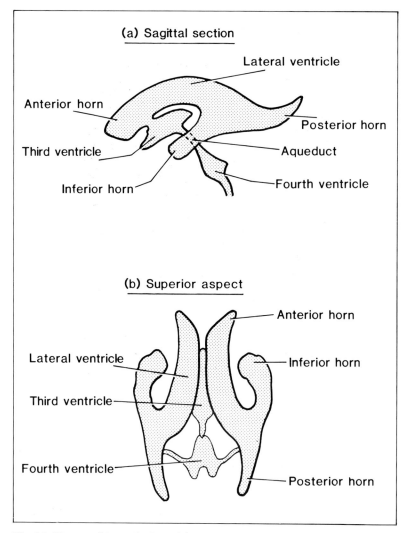

Fig. 6.1 Diagram of the cerebral ventricles.

hydrocephaly, whilst a block in any part of the ventricular system leads to obstructive hydrocephaly.

The easiest part of the ventricular system to visualise with ultrasound are the lateral ventricles. These are bilateral and have anterior, posterior and inferior horns. They contain the choroid plexus. The inferior horn is rarely seen in normal fetuses as it is lost in the echoes from the base of the skull.

The lateral ventricles are found by sliding the transducer slightly cephalad from the section required for BPD. Figure 6.2 illustrates both the anterior and posterior horns at approximately 18 weeks gestation.

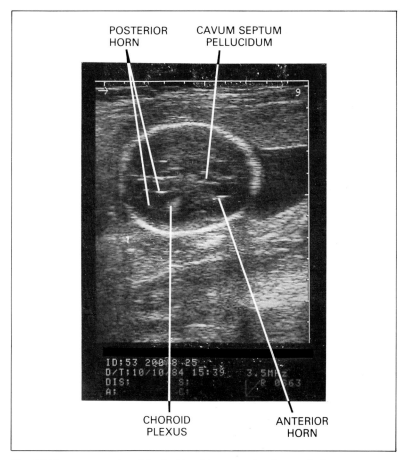

POSTERIOR HORN   CAVUM SEPTUM PELLUCIDUM

CHOROID PLEXUS   ANTERIOR HORN

Fig. 6.2 Transverse section of the fetal head demonstrating the ventricular system.

After 20 weeks both horns may not be visualised on the same section. Optimal views of the posterior horn are best obtained by sliding caudally from the section that demonstrates the anterior horns.

Figure 6.3 illustrates a pathological specimen of a fetal head at approximately the same level and demonstrates that ultrasound produces a very good representation of the anatomy.

Measurements of the ventricular system are expressed as anterior and posterior ventricular: hemisphere ratios. As can be appreciated from Figures 6.2 and 6.3 the anterior horn is a mere slit at this level. The measurement of the anterior horn is made from the midline to the lateral border of the ventricle but it is obvious that this is not the width of the anterior horn but its distance from the midline. The hemisphere is measured from the midline to the inner border of the skull in the same (lower) hemisphere. After 18 weeks gestation the anterior horn: hemisphere ratio (AVHR) should be less than 0.5. It is vital that the

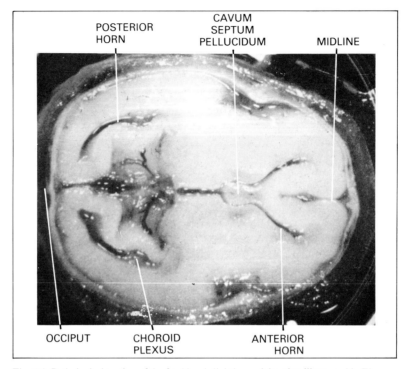

POSTERIOR HORN · CAVUM SEPTUM PELLUCIDUM · MIDLINE

OCCIPUT · CHOROID PLEXUS · ANTERIOR HORN

Fig. 6.3 Pathological section of the fetal head slightly caudal to that illustrated in Figure 6.2. Note how well the ultrasound reflects the anatomy.

section on which the AVH ratio is measured contains the cavum septum pellucidum and that the measurement of the anterior horn is taken anterior to this. The insula may be very prominent and may mimic the lateral border of the anterior horn (Fig. 6.4). Measurements of the AVH ratio that falsely use the insula will give high AVH ratios and allow wrong diagnoses of hydrocephaly to be made. The section on which the AVH ratio is measured must display both anterior horns and they must be symmetrical about the midline. The lower ventricle and hemisphere are measured as reverberation in the proximal hemisphere often obscures the margins of these structures.

The posterior horn has an easily appreciable width with a distinct medial border. The lateral border may not be clearly visualised so the lateral aspect of the choroid plexus may be taken as its outer limit (Fig. 6.2). The width of both the anterior and the posterior horn is expressed as a ratio over the cerebral hemisphere, and the normal range is illustrated in Figure 6.5.

The remainder of the ventricular system is not readily visualised in the normal fetus.

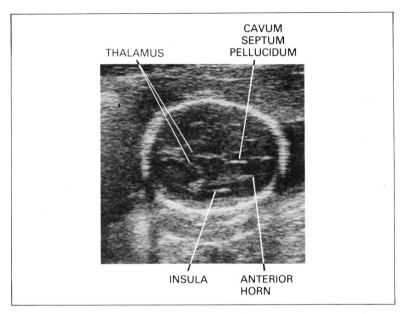

Fig. 6.4 Transverse section of the fetal head demonstrating the thalamus. Note also the insula and how easily this can be mistaken for the anterior horn of the lateral cerebral ventricle.

The thalamus and the hippocampus

The echo poor area between the ventricles is the thalamus (Fig. 6.6). Slight rotation of the transducer will now give a view of the hippocampus. This view is often obtained when searching for the correct section on which to measure the BPD or ventricles.

The posterior fossa

Further rotation of the transducer will now give a suboccipito-bregmatic view which will demonstrate the contents of the posterior fossa (Fig. 6.6). The most obvious structure is the dumb-bell shaped cerebellum which has two lateral lobes and a central connection known as the vermis. The fourth ventricle lies beneath the cerebellum but is not visible in normal fetuses. The space behind the cerebellum, and in front of the vault of the skull, is the cisterna magna. This is a reservoir for CSF.

THE FETAL FACE

Sliding the transducer caudally from the section on which the BPD should be measured will demonstrate the orbits. On a symmetrical

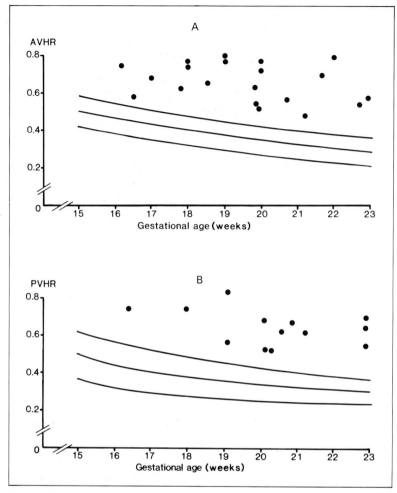

Fig. 6.5 Charts of the ventricular: hemisphere ratio. (a) Anterior horn (AVHR).
(b) Posterior horn (PVHR). The dots represent measurements obtained from
pathological proven cases of ventriculomegaly. (We are indebted to Professor Campbell
for permission to reproduce these charts.)

image (Fig. 6.7) the interocular distance, the binocular distance and the
orbital diameters may be measured. The ocular diameters should be
equal. Rotating the transducer to a plane at right angles to that used for
measuring the BPD will allow the soft tissues of the face to be
demonstrated. Sliding movements are necessary until the section shown
in Figure 6.8 is obtained. On this section the lens of the eye can often be
seen and the mouth will be seen. Profile views of the fetal face also
demonstrate soft tissue structures, but are particularly useful for
demonstrating the fetal nose and chin (Fig. 6.9).

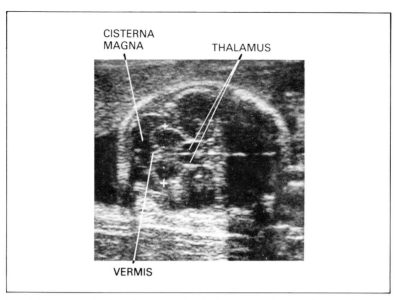

Fig. 6.6 The posterior fossa. The cerebellum is the structure between the two caliper markers which also demonstrate how the measurements of the transverse cerebellar diameter are obtained.

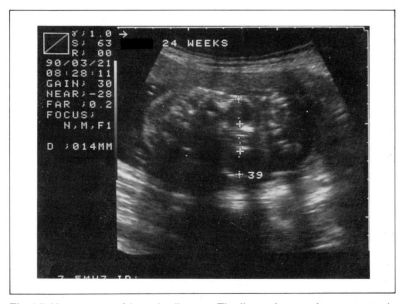

Fig. 6.7 Measurements of the ocular distances. The distance between the outer cursors is the binocular distance (39 mm) whilst that between the inner cursors is the interocular distance (14 mm). The ocular diameter is the distance from the outer cursor to the closer inner cursor.

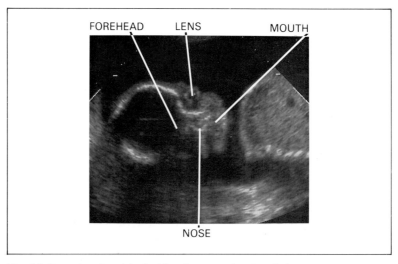

Fig. 6.8 Coronal section of the fetal face demonstrating the soft tissues.

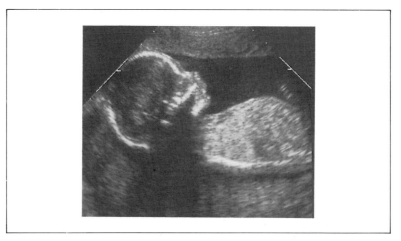

Fig. 6.9 Profile of the fetal face (mid-sagittal section) demonstrating a normal nose and chin.

A tangential view with the transducer angled up from beneath the fetal chin will demonstrate the lips and the nostrils (Fig. 6.10). The palate is best seen by returning to the view necessary for the measurement of the BPD and then sliding the transducer caudally past the level of the orbits. Careful study anteriorly will demonstrate fine movements of the fetal tongue. The very slightest move cephalad will now demonstrate the fetal palate (Fig. 6.11).

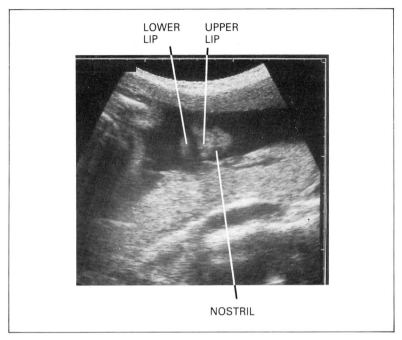

Fig. 6.10 Tangential view of the fetal face demonstrating lips and nostrils.

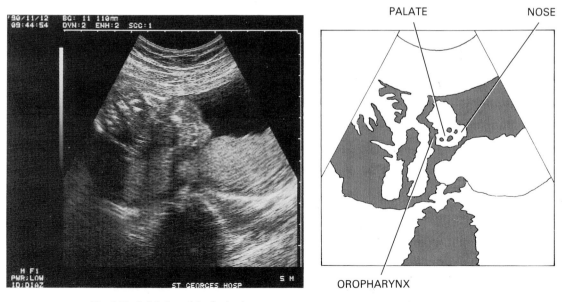

Fig. 6.11 Axial view of the fetal palate.

THE FETAL SPINE

The fetal spine is easily visualised because it produces high level echoes. Obtain a transverse section of the fetal body at any level. Now, slide the transducer around the maternal abdomen in order to bring the spine to the top of the screen. Rotating the transducer through 90° will now demonstrate the spine in longitudinal section together with the overlying skin covering. Particularly note the upsweep of the sacrum (Fig. 6.12). Rotating the transducer back through 90° will demonstrate the vertebrae in transverse section (Fig. 6.13). The entire length of the spine, i.e. every vertebra, should be examined in both sections. Care must be taken to stay at right angles to the long axis of the spine when examining it transversely so that the closed horseshoe or 'U' appearance of each vertebra is maintained — this is especially important when examining the sacrum. The spine is easily examined from 16 weeks gestation onwards, as long as the fetal position is favourable.

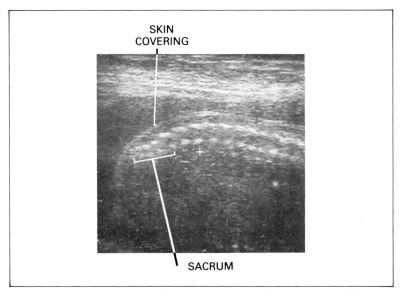

Fig. 6.12 Longitudinal section of the fetal spine demonstrating the up-sweep of the sacrum and the skin covering.

THE FETAL CHEST AND DIAPHRAGM

The ribs are readily recognised in both longitudinal and transverse section. Abnormalities of the ribs are rare although fusion may occur. The fetal clavicles are recognisable (Fig. 6.14).

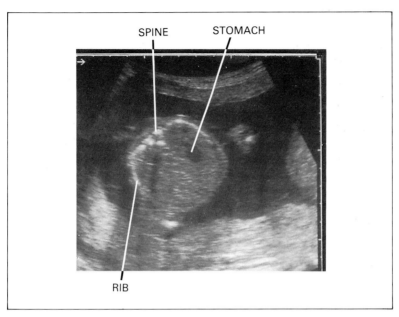

Fig. 6.13 Transverse section of the fetal abdomen demonstrating the 'U' shape of a normal vertebra.

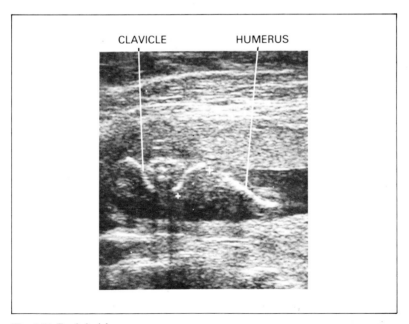

Fig. 6.14 Fetal clavicles.

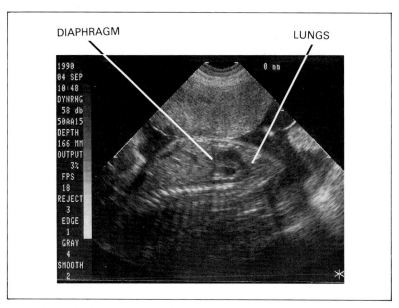

Fig. 6.15 Longitudinal section of the fetal body illustrating the diaphragm and lungs.

The most prominent structure in the chest is the fetal heart, which should occupy about one third of the cavity. The remainder of the chest is filled with the lungs, which produce homogeneous low level echoes (Fig. 6.15). In longitudinal section the diaphragm is recognisable (Fig. 6.15).

The normal anatomy of the fetal heart is illustrated in Figures 6.16–20. The right ventricle lies nearer the anterior chest wall and is characterised by the presence of the moderator band (Fig. 6.16). In the four chamber view, the two ventricles and the intraventricular septum are seen. Rotating the transducer slightly will demonstrate continuity between the ventricular septum and the aortic root (Fig. 6.17). Both atria are seen in the four chamber view and the flap of the foramen ovale may be seen in the left atrium (Fig. 6.16). Rotating the transducer together with caudal sliding movements will allow the arch of the aorta to be followed round to the descending thoracic aorta (Fig. 6.18). This view, which is known as the short axis view, demonstrates that the aorta is a tight shepherd's crook that appears to arise from the centre of the heart. The head and neck vessels can also clearly be seen.

Further rotation of the transducer now gives a transverse section of the root of the aorta surrounded by a much broader shepherd's crook that appears to arise from the anterior aspect of the heart (Fig. 6.19). This crook consists of the pulmonary trunk (arising from the right ventricle) and the ductus arteriosus which joins the descending aorta. In transverse section, at a level just cephalad to the four chamber view,

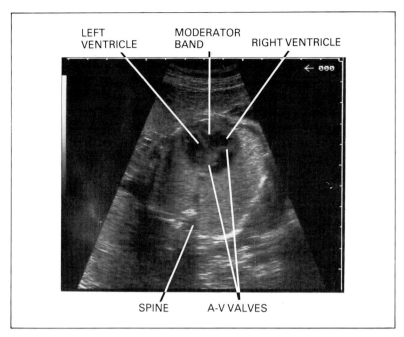

Fig. 6.16 Four chamber view of a normal fetal heart.

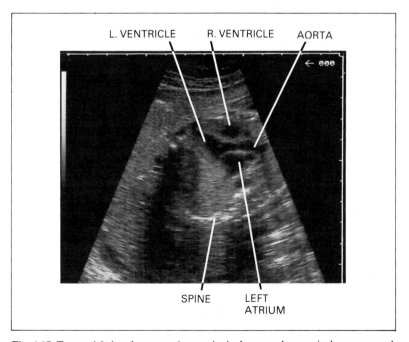

Fig. 6.17 Tangential view demonstrating continuity between the ventricular septum and the aortic root.

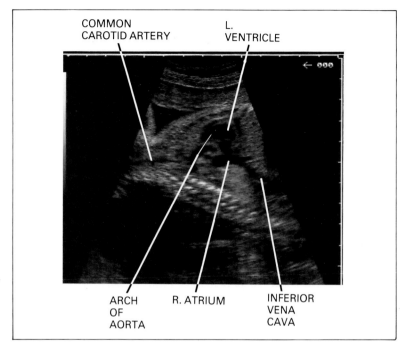

Fig. 6.18 The arch of the aorta. Note how it arises from the middle of the fetal heart (short axis view).

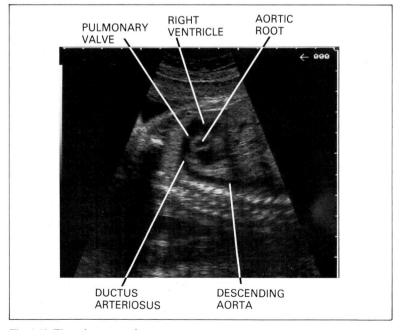

Fig. 6.19 The pulmonary arch.

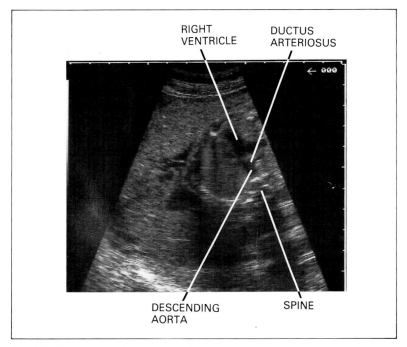

Fig. 6.20 Transverse section demonstrating the ductus arteriosus.

the ductus arteriosus is seen as a vessel running straight back to join the descending aorta (Fig. 6.20).

The fetal heart should have a regular beat, although it is not uncommon for it to slow down when the woman is scanned. This occurs more commonly if the woman lies flat on her back and the transducer is pressed firmly into her abdomen. The heart should rapidly return to a normal rate (120–160 beats per minute) on releasing the pressure. Study the heart for a few minutes looking for irregular beats. Finally, decide if the heart is in the left side of the fetal chest. Do not use the stomach as a landmark as, if the heart is in the right side of the chest (dextrocardia), it may be associated with a complete inversion of all the organs (situs inversus). You must orientate the fetal organs by using the presentation and the position of fetal spine.

Abnormalities of rhythm are best studied by use of the T-M mode. If the cursor of the M mode is placed through the origin of the aorta at the level of the valve, then the T-M mode will record the aortic valve which reflects the ventricular rate, together with the action of the right atrium (Fig. 6.21). If the fetal heart is in sinus rhythm there should be one atrial beat for every ventricular beat.

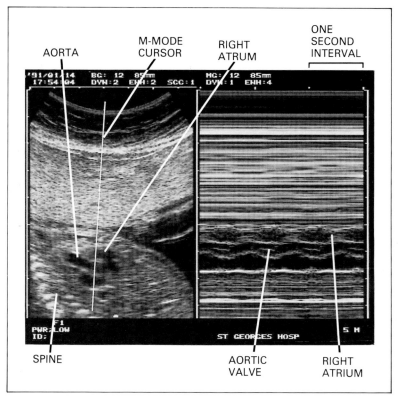

Fig. 6.21 The left hand image is a longitudinal view (short axis) of the fetal heart showing the position of the M-mode cursor. The right hand image demonstrates the M-mode. There is one aortic valve movement for each movement of the right atrium so the fetus is in sinus rhythm. The fetal heart rate can be determined by counting the number of aortic valve movements that occur in one second and multiplying by 60 (120 beats per minute in this example).

THE FETAL ABDOMEN

Obtain the view from which the AC measurement would be derived (see Ch. 5). A stomach bubble will be seen in the majority of fetuses after 16 weeks gestation. If no stomach bubble can be identified, rescanning in half an hour should demonstrate fluid in the stomach.

Slide caudally to the site of insertion of the umbilical cord and then rotate the transducer until a longitudinal section of the fetus is obtained, keeping the insertion in view. Note that the umbilical vein travels up through the liver at approximately 45°. Thus, if the section on which you intend to measure abdominal circumference has a long length of umbilical vein, you know you have an oblique section (Fig. 6.22). By careful rotation of the transducer at the site of insertion of the umbilical cord a transverse section of the cord, in the amniotic

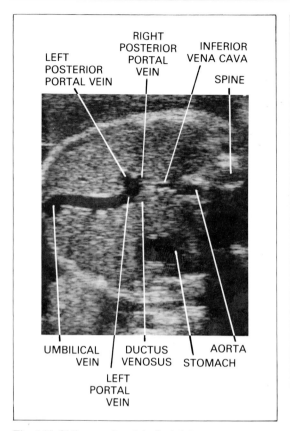

LEFT
POSTERIOR
PORTAL VEIN

RIGHT
POSTERIOR
PORTAL
VEIN

INFERIOR
VENA CAVA

SPINE

UMBILICAL
VEIN

DUCTUS
VENOSUS

AORTA

STOMACH

LEFT
PORTAL
VEIN

Fig. 6.22 Oblique section of the fetal abdomen demonstrating the course of the umbilical and portal veins.

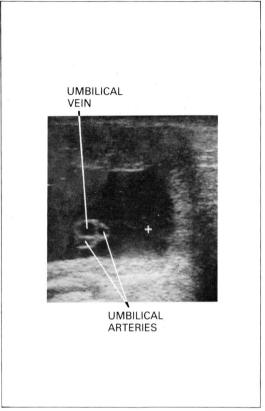

UMBILICAL
VEIN

UMBILICAL
ARTERIES

Fig. 6.23 Transverse section of the umbilical cord.

fluid, is obtained. It should contain three vessels: two arteries and a vein (Fig. 6.23).

Return now to a transverse section of the fetal abdomen and follow the umbilical vein into the liver. It joins with the left portal vein, which enters a cruciate arrangement consisting of itself, its two branches and the ductus venosus (Fig. 6.22). Most of the blood that is being returned to the fetus from the placenta passes through the ductus venosus to the right atrium by way of the inferior vena cava. The gallbladder may also be visualised on a cross-sectional view of the fetal abdomen (Fig. 6.27). Note the tiny rim of free fluid that is often seen between the liver and the abdominal wall.

Study the bowel in both longitudinal and cross section. Late in the third trimester the colon may be very obvious as sonolucent areas around the periphery of the abdominal cavity (Fig. 6.24). The remainder of bowel is usually barely distinguishable.

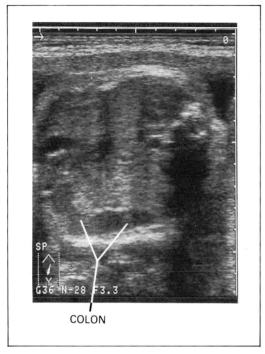

Fig. 6.24 Transverse section of the fetal abdomen at 32 weeks gestation demonstrating the appearances of the normal colon.

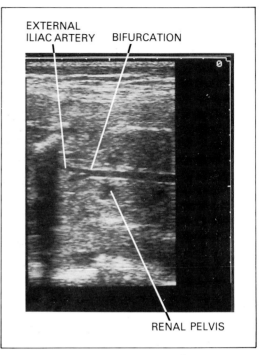

Fig. 6.25 Longitudinal section of the fetal abdomen demonstrating the iliac bifurcation of the aorta.

Now return to a longitudinal section of the fetal abdomen and locate the fetal aorta. It can be followed down to the iliac bifurcation and into the leg as the femoral artery (Fig. 6.25). Alongside the aorta, in the upper abdomen, the inferior vena cava is visible (Fig. 6.26). Note that this passes through the diaphragm and can be seen entering the right atrium. The aorta passes behind the diaphragm.

The fetal spleen may be seen on the left of the abdominal cavity in the third trimester.

THE FETAL URINARY TRACT

The fetal bladder is usually readily visible in both transverse and longitudinal sections of the fetal abdomen and pelvis. Prior to 16 weeks gestation it may be empty for periods of up to 45 minutes. Its volume can be calculated by obtaining the maximum longitudinal (L), transverse (T) and anteroposterior (AP) diameters (cm) and multiplying them by 0.5233 (see Ch. 2 for explanation). If the process is repeated 15 minutes later then the increase in volume multiplied by four will give

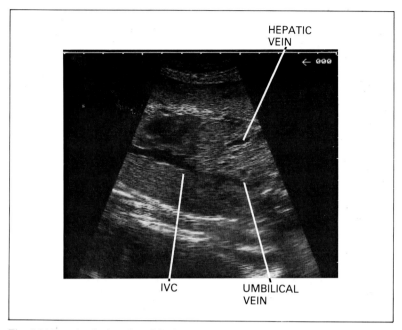

Fig. 6.26 Longitudinal section of the fetal abdomen demonstrating the course of the inferior vena cava.

the hourly fetal urinary production rate (HFUPR). If the volume has decreased over the 15 minute period, it is necessary to repeat the measurement 15 minutes later.

The fetal kidneys may be seen from 14 weeks gestation and are easily visible by 20 weeks. Most observers identify them initially in a transverse section of the abdomen. By sliding caudally from the section required for measurement of the AC, look closely in the para-spinal gutters. The first clue that you have found the kidney is the echo free area that represents the renal pelvis (Fig. 6.27). If the fetal spine is directly anterior then both kidneys may be seen on the same section. If the spine is lateral then the lower kidney is usually hidden in the acoustic shadow from the spine. In order to see it the transducer should be rotated around the maternal abdomen in an attempt to bring the spine to the top of the screen.

Having located the kidneys in the transverse plane, alter the transducer such that one kidney is in the centre of the screen. Rotate the transducer through 90° keeping that kidney in view until a longitudinal section is obtained (Fig. 6.28). If the upper and lower limits of the kidney are difficult to see, make tiny lateral sliding movements. If the fetus should breathe then the limits are usually well demarcated. Note the appearance of the renal pelvis in this view. After 24–26 weeks marked fetal lobulations may be seen (Fig. 6.28). The

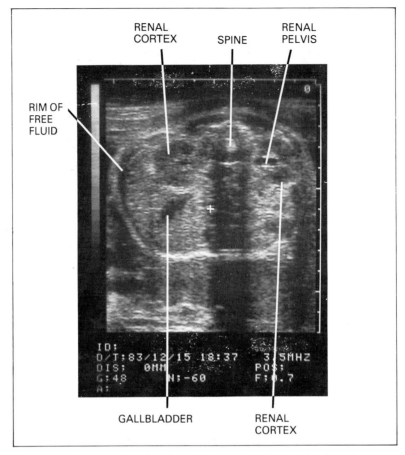

Fig. 6.27 Transverse section of the fetal abdomen at 30 weeks gestation demonstrating the kidneys. Note how the acoustic shadow of the spine hides the umbilical vein.

echogenicity of the kidney is very similar to that of the fetal lungs, i.e. low level, homogeneous echoes.

The following measurements of the kidney can be made. In transverse section, measure the maximum transverse and anteroposterior diameter of both the kidney and the renal pelvis. In the normal fetus the renal pelvis may measure up to one third of the diameter of the kidney. Measurement of the maximum thickness of the renal cortex is also made in this view (Fig. 6.30). Finally, measure the longitudinal length of the kidney. Charts showing normal values for these parameters are shown in Figures 6.29 (a,b,c) and 8.21.

The adrenal glands are located at the upper pole of the kidney and may occasionally be recognised from 20 weeks gestation onwards. Their main interest, ultrasonically, lies in the ability to mimic an absent kidney (see Ch. 8).

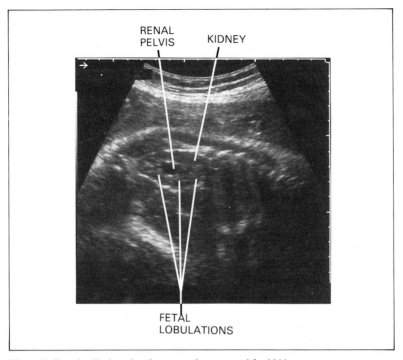

RENAL
PELVIS   KIDNEY

FETAL
LOBULATIONS

Fig. 6.28 Longitudinal section demonstrating a normal fetal kidney.

THE FETAL GENDER

It is possible to determine the sex of the fetus from 14 weeks onwards. The diagnosis depends upon the fetus having its legs apart and on recognising the characteristic echo pattern from both males and females. You should not make the diagnosis unless you are absolutely certain; do not diagnose a female by an apparent lack of male parts. Apart from parental interest, fetal gender is important in women who are carriers of sex-linked conditions such as haemophilia. In these conditions only the male fetus is affected.

Figure 6.31 illustrates a male fetus at 20 weeks. The penis is visible but care should be taken not to confuse loops of umbilical cord for the penis. Figure 6.32 illustrates the scrotum of a fetus at 32 weeks. Figure 6.33a demonstrates the echo pattern from female genitalia at 24 weeks, whilst Figure 6.33b is at 33 weeks.

Parents seem to be equally divided as to whether they wish to know the sex of their fetus. We suggest that you should never ask the parents if they wish to know the sex of their baby, but if they want to know you should try to tell them. Asking the parents seems to put them under pressure to make a decision one way or the other, and many parents assume that if you have asked the question the fetus must be a male.

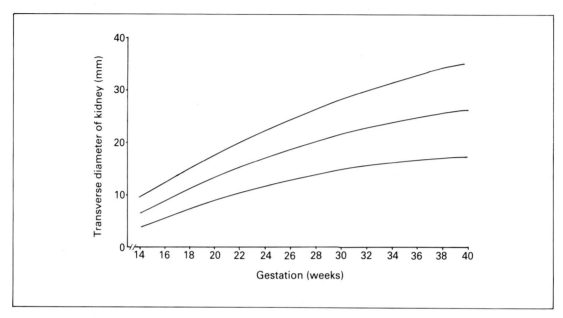

Fig. 6.29 (a) Growth of the transverse diameter (T) of the kidney with gestational age.

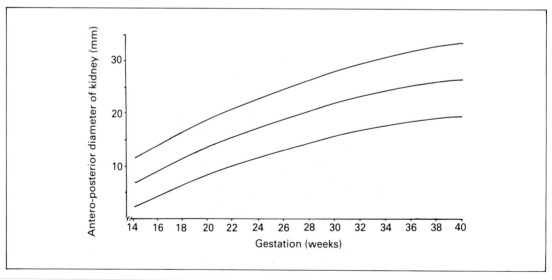

(b) Growth of the anteroposterior diameter (AP) of the kidney with gestational age.

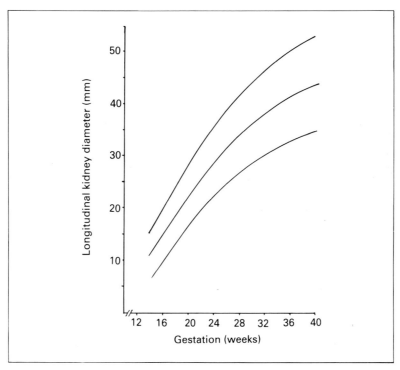

(c) Growth of the longitudinal diameter (L) with gestational age. (Mean ± 2 SDs.)

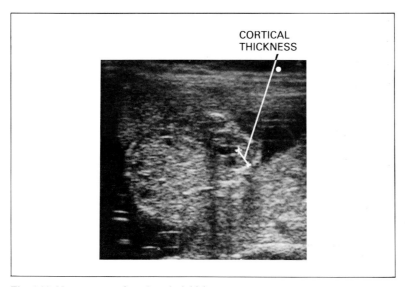

Fig. 6.30 Measurement of renal cortical thickness.

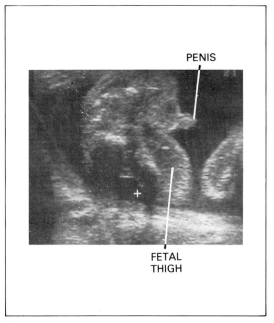

Fig. 6.31 Male genitalia at 20 weeks gestation.

Fig. 6.32 Male genitalia at 32 weeks gestation.

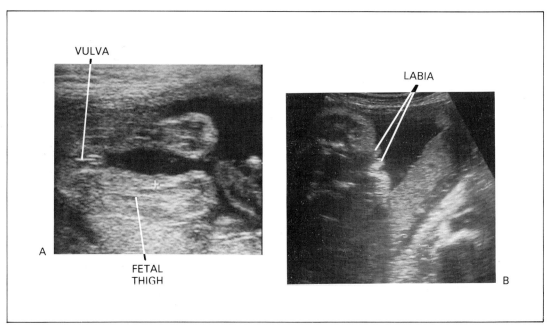

Fig. 6.33 Female genitalia at (a) 24 weeks gestation, and (b) 33 weeks gestation.

Never guess; if you are unsure, say you do not know. It's costly repainting the nursery and changing all the baby clothes from blue to pink!

THE FETAL LIMBS

Chapter 5 describes how to obtain measurements of the fetal femur. Commonly this is the only long bone measured although a visual assessment of the other long bones should be made. Normal values for all the long bones are available (Appendix 5). The tibia and fibula may be measured together (Fig. 6.34). They are best found by obtaining a transverse view of the abdomen and sliding the transducer caudally. The lower end of the femur (at the knee) is usually seen and then by rotation the lower leg may be demonstrated. You should ensure that both bones are visualised but generally only the tibia is measured.

To measure the arm bones a transverse section of the chest is obtained and the transducer is moved cephalad until one humerus is seen in cross-section. Rotation of the transducer will then demonstrate the full length of the humerus (Fig. 6.35). Care should be taken as the end of the humerus may be difficult to define because of acoustic shadowing from the fetal ribs, especially with the lower arm which may

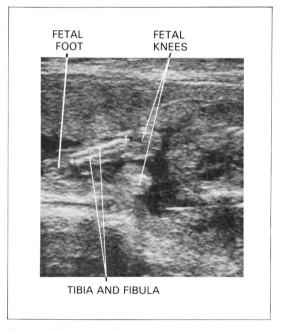

Fig. 6.34 The tibia and fibula at 19 weeks gestation.

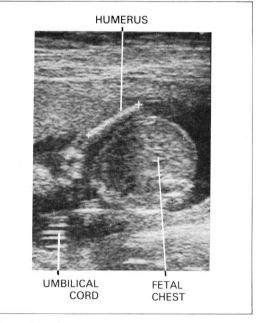

Fig. 6.35 The humerus at 19 weeks gestation.

be between the fetal body and the placenta. Sliding the transducer to the fetal elbow will now demonstrate two bright echoes which are the radius and ulna in cross-section. Again, rotation of the transducer will produce a view of the entire length of the complex. The radius and ulna should be visualised together (Fig. 6.36) but commonly only the radius is measured.

Finally, study the fetal hands and feet. They are found by following the arm or leg to its limit. It is necessary to learn to appreciate the angle of the foot to the leg so that talipes may be recognised. Fetal activity may make it difficult but you should attempt to get a view of the feet that allows you to count the toes. Ideally, this should be the view that would give a foot print so that the metatarsal bones can also be seen. Counting fingers is also difficult as the fetus often has a closed fist. Patience is necessary but again you should try to demonstrate the metacarpal bones and to appreciate the normal position of the hand to the forearm (Fig. 6.37).

Having examined the fetus as above you can be sure that nothing major will go unnoticed. When you have learnt to recognise the normal anatomy you will quickly become aware that 'something is wrong'. As there are a limited number of faults in any one fetal organ, making the definitive diagnosis is largely a process of exclusion.

EARLY ASSESSMENT OF FETAL ANATOMY

The use of transvaginal probes now enables some of the fetal anatomy to be studied in the first trimester and hence fetal anomalies can now be

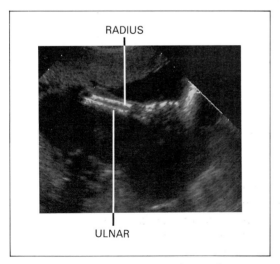

Fig. 6.36 The radius and ulna at 19 weeks gestation.

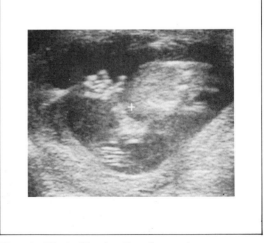

Fig. 6.37 The fetal hand at 15 weeks gestation.

detected at this stage. For example, from 9–10 weeks gestation, major abnormalities such as anencephaly, spina bifida and encephalocoele may be diagnosed.

Systematic examination of the fetal anatomy at these early gestations is often limited by the fetal position and the restricted manoeuvrability of the transvaginal probe. These two factors limit its potential as a method of routine screening. If, however, you regularly use a transvaginal probe to assess early pregnancy, you should familiarise yourself with the anatomy that is visible and how it changes with increasing gestation. For instance it is normal for every fetus to have an 'omphalocoele' at 8 weeks gestation. Diagnosis in early pregnancy will allow vaginal termination but the above problems mean that, in the foreseeable future, it is unlikely to replace the routine 18–20 week scan.

WHICH FETUSES SHOULD HAVE ANOMALY SCANS?

An ultrasound examination is in the unique position of being both a screening test and a diagnostic test for fetal anomalies. Table 6.1 indicates those women who should have a high resolution ultrasound scan as a diagnostic test. Ultrasound in these cases must only be performed by people who have been trained to detect abnormalities.

Table 6.1 Indications for high resolution ultrasound examination

Raised MSAFP
Low MSAFP or positive triple test
Women undergoing amniocentesis
Women who have had chorion villus sampling
Women with a personal or family history of anomaly
Women with a personal or family history of a chromosome anomaly that has a structural marker
Oligohydramnios
Polyhydramnios
Maternal diabetes mellitus
Women in preterm labour especially if the presentation is breech
Multiple gestation
Women exposed to potential teratogens in early pregnancy
Women with suspicious findings on routine ultrasound
Women with symmetrically small fetuses

In our opinion it is not reasonable to expect all fetal abnormalities to be diagnosed at a routine ultrasound examination. If the approach in Chapter 5 is followed then no major structural abnormality should be missed. For instance anencephaly should not be missed. It is also unreasonable to overlook large protruding masses such as encephalocoele, cystic hygroma and abdominal wall defects. If the ventricular: hemisphere ratio is routinely measured then most cases of hydrocephaly should also be detected at 16–20 weeks. Abnormal fluid collections such as ascites and pleural effusion should not be overlooked, and severe oligohydramnios or polyhydramnios should also be recognised.

It is unreasonable to expect the ultrasonographer to diagnose all renal lesions, or cardiac lesions, and when such diagnoses are made they should be viewed as a bonus. Other abnormalities, such as microcephaly, may also be difficult to recognise. It is our opinion that no blame should be attached to an ultrasonographer who fails to diagnose lesions such as microcephaly which may only be diagnosable by serial measurements. If, however, there is a discrepancy between the BPD and the femur length, the woman should be referred for a detailed scan so that microcephaly or dwarfism may be excluded.

CHAPTER SEVEN
Cranio-spinal defects

One in 50 babies born in the United Kingdom are born with a congenital abnormality, and in one in 100 this will be a major abnormality. Neural tube defects (NTD) account for half of the major anomalies and have an incidence that varies from 2–5 per 1000 births. The cause of NTDs is unknown but it is currently thought to be related to a relative deficiency in folic acid in the mother. The two commonest forms of NTD are spina bifida and anencephaly, and they are equal in occurrence.

Anencephaly (absence of the cranial vault) is not compatible with life so prenatal diagnosis is desirable. We feel that prenatal diagnosis is also desirable in cases of spina bifida as only about half of the infants with open spina bifida will survive five years and the vast majority of the survivors have major degrees of handicap. As more than 90% of infants born with NTD are born to patients who have not had a previously affected child a screening test is necessary. This is available by estimation of maternal serum alphafetoprotein.

ALPHAFETOPROTEIN (AFP)

AFP is virtually undetectable in the adult but is easily detectable in embryonic and fetal life. It is a protein which the embryo produces from the yolk sac and the fetus produces from its liver. In the normal fetus the AFP is excreted into the amniotic fluid via fetal urine and crosses the placenta to enter the mother's blood.

The level of AFP in the fetal blood reaches a peak at 16–18 weeks gestation and this is reflected in the levels of AFP in the amniotic fluid. In maternal blood AFP continues to increase in concentration until 32 weeks, probably due to increasing placental permeability.

Most laboratories report the maternal serum AFP (MSAFP) levels in multiples of the median (MoM) as this seems to lessen laboratory error.

123

As MSAFP is not a perfect screening test it is necessary to set the upper limit of normal to a level that will not include too many normal pregnant women. This has been accepted to be 2.5 × MoM. About 2 per 100 women will have a MSAFP value above this level. In areas where the incidence of NTDs is 2–3 per 1000 births the chances of a woman with a MSAFP greater than 2.5 × MoM having a fetus with a NTD are about 1 in 20. Having a normal MSAFP is not a guarantee that the fetus does not have a NTD as a MSAFP above 2.5 × MoM will only detect about 85% of cases of open spina bifida.

A woman who has had a child or fetus with a NTD has a 1 in 20 chance of recurrence. If she has had two affected infants the chances are increased to 1 in 10. A normal MSAFP is not adequate reassurance in these cases and the women should have a detailed ultrasound examination.

What to do with a woman with a raised MSAFP

Table 7.1 lists the causes of raised MSAFP. The test should be repeated and a simple ultrasound examination should be performed. This should accurately establish the gestational age and exclude twins or anencephaly as a cause.

Table 7.1 Causes of raised MSAFP

Laboratory error
Idiopathic

Diagnosable by simple ultrasound
Wrong gestational age
Multiple pregnancy
Hydatidiform mole
Intrauterine death
Anencephaly

Diagnosable by high resolution ultrasound
Spina bifida
Omphalocoele/gastroschisis
Obstructive uropathies
Oesophageal atresia

Diagnosable by fetal bladder puncture
Finnish type congenital nephrosis★

★ The urine AFP is very raised in these cases

There are then two possible ways of managing the woman: amniocentesis or high resolution ultrasound.

Amniocentesis is performed in many cases in order to estimate the AFP in the amniotic fluid. If this is raised (and if there is a second band of acetylcholinesterase on electrophoresis) the woman is usually offered a termination of pregnancy. This approach has two main disadvantages:

1. Amniocentesis carries a small risk of causing a miscarriage (see

Ch. 9). In about 19 per 20 cases of raised MSAFP the fetus will be normal, so for every five cases of neural tube defect detected by amniocentesis one normal pregnancy will be lost.

2. There is a small false positive rate associated with this method (about 1 in 400). That is, occasionally a normal fetus may be aborted.

The alternative method is to perform a detailed, high resolution ultrasound examination. In skilled hands it should be possible to decide if the fetus is abnormal, to specify the type of anomaly and to say how extensive it appears. Although there will be a few cases in which a small abnormality will be missed, the false positive rate should be the same or less than that of amniocentesis and studies of amniotic fluid AFP. The method that involves ultrasound does not carry the risk of the amniocentesis and has the added advantage of being able to visualise the abnormality such that a prognosis may be given.

HOW TO LOOK FOR SPECIFIC ANOMALIES

Anencephaly

Absence of the cranial vault is readily detected from 14 weeks gestation onwards. Figure 7.1 illustrates the usual appearance. Most observers are initially struck by the 'frog's eye' appearance of the fetus. Although it is unreasonable to expect all anomalies to be detected at a routine ultrasound clinic, this is a diagnosis which should not be overlooked after 14 weeks gestation. The commonest reason for missing the diagnosis is that the fetal head cannot be visualised and is assumed to be deep in the maternal pelvis. Such women should always be asked to fill

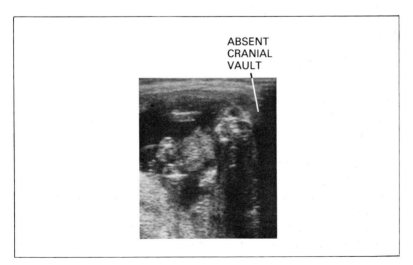

Fig. 7.1 An anencephalic fetus. Note the typical frog's eye appearance.

their bladders and should be tipped head down. If the fetal position is still not favourable, bring the woman back a week later; do not confirm gestational age by measurement of the femur and send her away.

Spina bifida

Spina bifida refers to the bony defect alone (Fig. 7.2). It is the accompanying disruption of the nervous tissue of the spinal cord that causes the paralysis. This disturbance of the nerves is not fully developed until the nerves are exposed to air, i.e. not until after delivery. This means that the fetus with spina bifida (or anencephaly) will empty its bladder and kick. Never, never say an 'at risk' fetus is normal because it is moving its legs.

The method for scanning the normal spine is described in Chapter 6. Before a spine can be passed as normal you must have examined every vertebra in both transverse and longitudinal section. Figure 7.3 illustrates a cross-section of a fetal spine with a meningocoele. Note the 'V' shape of the echoes from the vertebra rather than the normal 'U' shape. In this case the discrete sac of the meningocoele makes the diagnosis relatively simple. Figure 7.4 illustrates a meningomyelocoele. Nervous tissue can be seen well outside the spinal canal.

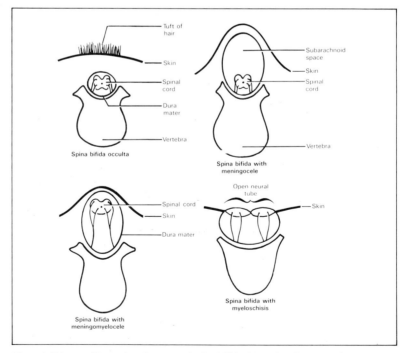

Fig. 7.2 Diagram illustrating the types of spina bifida. Note that the term spina bifida strictly only refers to the bony defect.

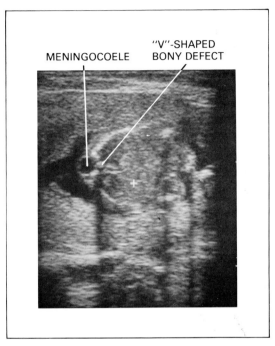

MENINGOCOELE   "V"-SHAPED BONY DEFECT

Fig. 7.3 Transverse section of a fetal abdomen demonstrating a meningocoele. Careful examination of the sac failed to demonstrate nervous tissue strands within the sac.

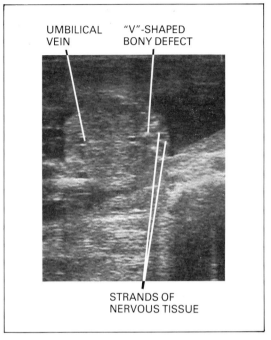

UMBILICAL VEIN   "V"-SHAPED BONY DEFECT

STRANDS OF NERVOUS TISSUE

Fig. 7.4 Transverse section of the fetal spine demonstrating a meningomyelocoele. The sac contains obvious strands of nervous tissue.

In longitudinal section a break in the skin covering may be the only clue. It is not always possible to obtain an adequate longitudinal view, especially if the fetal spine is posterior, and in such cases detailed study of the transverse sections may also be impossible. If you are unsure, always bring the woman back. Occasionally, a direct dorsal (anteroposterior) view will demonstrate the sac of a meningocoele or a separation of the line of the ossification centres. Normality of the spine should not be determined by use of this view alone, transverse sections should always be studied. Figure 7.5 illustrates an apparently normal spine in longitudinal view, but a slight sideways movement demonstrates a defect (Fig. 7.6), which is more clearly seen in transverse view (Fig. 7.7).

Hydrocephaly

Often the first clue to the presence of spina bifida is hydrocephaly (Fig. 7.8). Hydrocephaly (or ventriculomegaly) occurs in about 80% of fetuses with spina bifida. It makes the prognosis much worse as mental retardation is more common if both conditions are present.

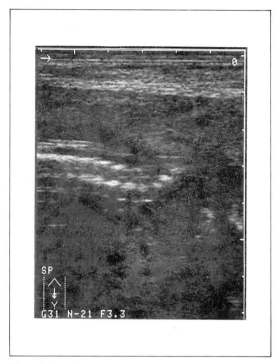

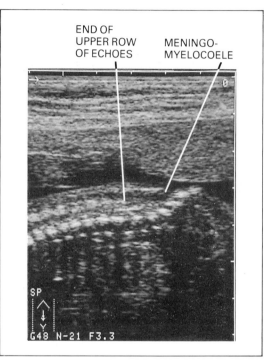

Fig. 7.5 Longitudinal scan of lower spine and sacrum demonstrating an apparently normal spine.

Fig. 7.6 Slight lateral movement from Figure 7.5 demonstrates a break in the line of echoes from the spine.

The method of measuring the ventricles is described in Chapter 6. The results of both the anterior horn: cerebral hemisphere ratio (AVHR) and the posterior horn: hemisphere ratio (PVHR) should be plotted on the appropriate charts. Figure 6.5 illustrates the charts for the AVHR and the PVHR with several pathological cases plotted upon it. The difference between the normals and abnormals is clear-cut in the vast majority of cases.

The AVHR is simple to measure and should be measured on all fetuses in the second trimester.

The diagnosis of hydrocephaly is made on the ventricular: hemisphere ratios; it is not made on the presence or absence of a large head. Although hydrocephalics may develop a large head in late pregnancy, the BPD and HC are commonly reduced in comparison to the femur and AC in cases of spina bifida with hydrocephaly in early pregnancy. Indeed, if the BPD and HC are found to be small in comparison to the femur, this should prompt a careful search for spina bifida (or microcephaly).

Hydrocephaly may occur in the absence of spina bifida; this is known as isolated hydrocephaly. This tends to be more severe than hydrocephaly associated with spina bifida. The recurrence risks for

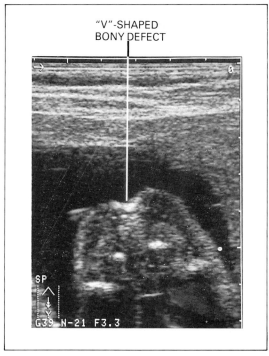

"V"-SHAPED
BONY DEFECT

Fig. 7.7 Transverse section of the spine in Figures 7.5 and 7.6 — at approximately the level of the second sacral vertebra — demonstrating the now obvious bony defect of spina bifida.

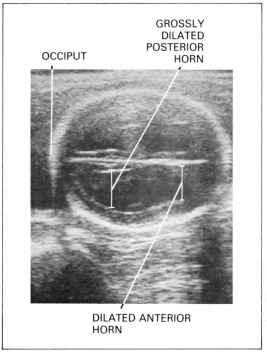

OCCIPUT

GROSSLY
DILATED
POSTERIOR
HORN

DILATED ANTERIOR
HORN

Fig. 7.8 Transverse section of the fetal head demonstrating hydrocephaly. The AVHR is 0.8 and the PVHR is 0.9. This was associated with a large lumbosacral meningomyelocoele.

isolated hydrocephaly are about 1 in 30 unless it is the rarer type due to sex-linked aqueduct stenosis which carries a recurrence risk of 1 in 4. This means that if you are scanning a woman who has had a previous male infant with hydrocephaly you should perform serial scans in the present pregnancy until 26 weeks (as aqueduct stenosis may present late) or until you are sure that it is a female fetus.

Other cranial signs associated with spina bifida

Recently, abnormal head shapes have been described in association with spina bifida. The fetal head, at the level on which the BPD is measured, should be the shape of a rugby ball (Fig. 5.2). Blunting of the sinciput, known as the lemon sign (Fig. 7.9), should arouse suspicion of a co-existent spina bifida.

The lemon sign may suggest the presence of spina bifida, but care should be taken that the view obtained is exactly at the level on which the BPD would be measured (Fig. 5.2) as slight malrotation of the transducer may include a view of the superior aspects of the orbits, giving a false lemon sign.

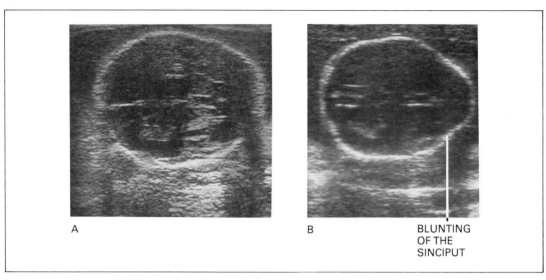

A

B

BLUNTING
OF THE
SINCIPUT

Fig. 7.9 Transverse sections of the fetal head at the level of the lateral ventricles.
(a) Normal fetus. (b) Fetus with spina bifida demonstrating the lemon sign. Note that
the lateral cerebral ventricles are not dilated.

The normal cerebellum is dumb-bell shaped (Fig. 6.6) but in many
cases of spina bifida the contents of the posterior fossa may be prolapsed
giving rise to a banana shaped cerebellum. This is known as the
Arnold–Chiari malformation.

Very rarely, a fetus with a meningomyelocoele and associated
hydrocephaly may appear to have an empty posterior fossa because of
the Arnold–Chiari malformation. In these cases the medulla oblongata
and the cerebellum are displaced caudally and cannot be identified
ultrasonically.

Encephalocoele

This is a rare form of NTD which may be thought of as a high spina
bifida. There is a bony defect in the cranial vault, usually in the occiput
(although it may be in the frontal, nasal or parietal bones) through
which protrudes a sac composed of dura mater. In most cases the sac
contains parts of the brain and prognosis is poor (Fig. 7.10). Very
rarely, the sac may contain only CSF in which case it is referred to as an
occipital meningocoele and has a good prognosis (Fig. 7.11).

Encephalocoeles are usually isolated lesions but occasionally they
may be associated with polycystic kidneys and polydactyly; this is
known as Meckel's syndrome. This is an autosomal recessive condition
and so has a 1 in 4 chance of recurrence. The recurrence rate for the
isolated condition is 1 in 20.

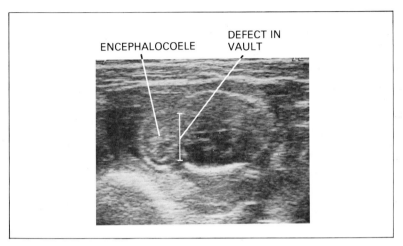

Fig. 7.10 Transverse section of the fetal head demonstrating an encephalocoele that contains most of the contents of the posterior fossa.

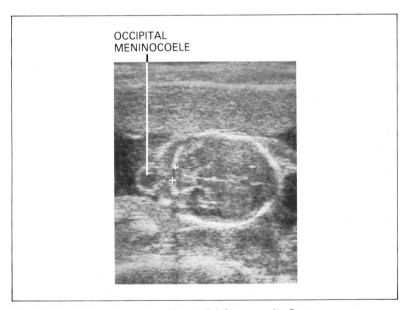

Fig. 7.11 Occipital meningocoele with a skull defect measuring 7 mm.

Microcephaly

Microcephaly means a small brain enclosed within a small skull. It is not a neural tube defect. Many microcephalics die soon after birth and those that survive are not only severely mentally retarded but are also dwarfed.

Microcephaly may be caused by virus infections (especially rubella), irradiation, maternal heroin addiction and some drugs. A few cases are associated with an autosomal recessive mode of inheritance. In most cases the cause is never established.

Ultrasound diagnosis of microcephaly may not be easy. Some cases undoubtedly develop late in pregnancy and will not, therefore, be detected on routine early ultrasound examination. Furthermore, it is not a structural abnormality but a severe slowing of the growth rate of the fetal head. This calls for careful, serial measurements of all growth parameters starting as early in the pregnancy as possible. Ideally, dates should be established by an early estimation of crown–rump length. Serial measurements involve BPD, HC, AC, and femur length and the H:A ratio. Figure 7.12 illustrates a typical case. The poor head growth leads to a decline in the H:A ratio but the diagnosis in this case could not be made with certainty until 24 weeks.

The diagnosis of microcephaly is best made by serial measurements which demonstrate poor head growth despite normal growth of the fetal

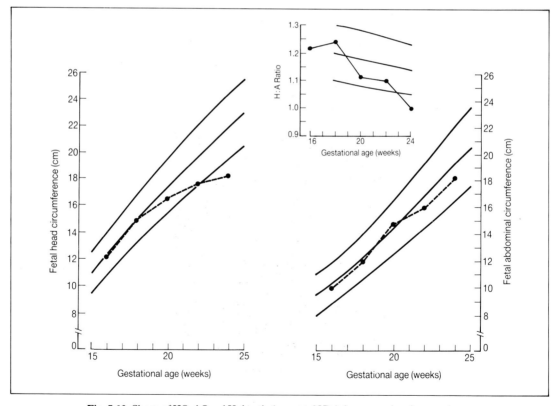

Fig. 7.12 Charts of HC, AC and H:A ratio (mean ± 2SDs) demonstrating the growth pattern in a case of microcephaly.

femur and abdominal girth. Diagnosis from a single measurement should only be made if the BPD and HC are more than three standard deviations below the mean, whilst other fetal parameters are of normal size.

The diagnosis is usually not made until after 20 weeks. It may be that the diagnosis will not become apparent until after the gestation at which the referring clinician is prepared to terminate the pregnancy. Careful discussion is needed to decide at what gestation serial scans should cease.

Rare abnormalities

Hydranencephaly is a congenital absence of the cerebral hemispheres and is recognised by the complete absence of echoes from within the cerebral vault. Theoretically, it is possible to distinguish it from severe obstructive hydrocephaly because in the latter case the middle cerebral artery can be seen pulsating at the site of the Sylvian fissure. As hydranencephaly is due to bilateral carotid occlusion, no pulsations are seen. Distinguishing between the conditions is academic as both have a very poor prognosis.

There is a group of conditions known collectively as the *arrhinencephaly–holoprosencephaly/cyclops syndrome*. They all involve a

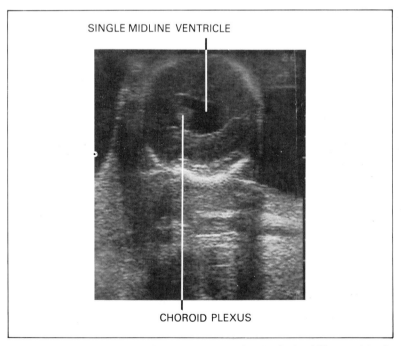

SINGLE MIDLINE VENTRICLE

CHOROID PLEXUS

Fig. 7.13 Oblique section of the fetal head demonstrating the single midline ventricle of holoprosencephaly.

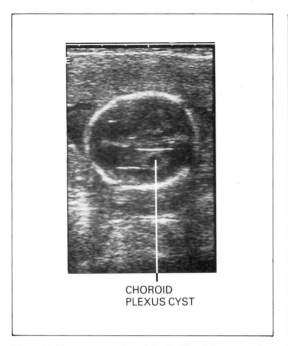

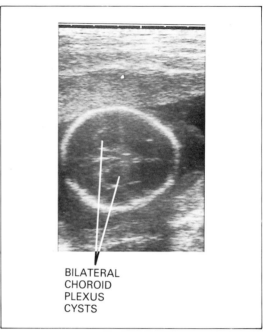

Fig. 7.14 Transverse section of the fetal head demonstrating a small choroid plexus cyst. There may also be a small cyst in the upper hemisphere but reverberation prevents adequate imaging.

Fig. 7.15 Transverse section of the fetal head demonstrating large, bilateral choroid plexus cysts.

midline fusion defect such that in the most severe case, holoprosencephaly, there is only a single midline cerebral ventricle (Fig. 7.13). Less severe cases may involve only absence of the cavum septum pellucidum. They are commonly associated with cyclops or median cleft lips.

The choroid plexus may demonstrate small cysts, up to about 10 mm in diameter, in early pregnancy (Fig. 7.14). They are often bilateral although reverberation may prevent the cyst in the proximal hemisphere from being visualised. They are thought to be developmental and usually resolve by 24 weeks gestation with no residual problems. Large cysts of the choroid plexus that fill the lateral ventricle (Fig. 7.15) or cysts that are not resolving by 22 weeks gestation may be associated with chromosome abnormalities. The fetus should be thoroughly examined looking for other structural markers (Appendix 3) and if present, then karyotyping should be offered. Choroid plexus cysts should not be confused with hydrocephaly or porencephalic cysts. The latter are cysts found in the cerebral hemisphere and are the result of liquefaction of an intracranial haemorrhage. The most common cause is hypoxic rupture of the small

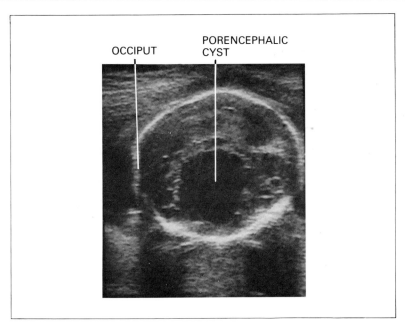

Fig. 7.16 Oblique section through the fetal head demonstrating a very large porencephalic cyst.

vessels of the germinal matrix that surround the ventricles. They are distinguishable from choroid plexus cysts because they extend from the ventricle into the cerebral hemisphere and are usually unilateral (Fig. 7.16). The prognosis depends upon the size and the location, but it is generally grave.

Abnormalities of the posterior fossa are very rare but often have a terrible prognosis. Many are associated with chromosome anomalies. The most common is absence of all or part of the cerebellum. Distension of the fourth cerebral ventricle — the Dandy–Walker syndrome (Fig. 7.17) — is an obstructive form of hydrocephaly with a poor prognosis.

Abnormalities in the shape of the fetal skull may be diagnosed by ultrasound. The experienced ultrasonographer will be aware of the long, narrow head (dolichocephaly) that the fetus presenting by the breech may have. Craniostenosis is a very rare condition in which the skull sutures fuse prematurely, and is diagnosable ultrasonically. In these cases the cephalic index may be useful (see Ch. 5). In dolichocephaly the index is reduced and in brachycephaly it is increased. In craniostenosis, the BPD and the cephalic index are persistently low.

Sacral agenesis (caudal regression syndrome) is an extremely rare abnormality that is almost exclusively seen in infants born to mothers

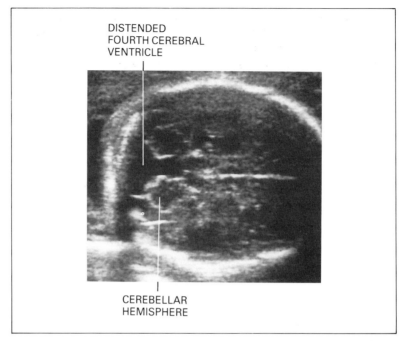

Fig. 7.17 Occipitobregmatic view of the posterior fossa demonstrating a Dandy–Walker cyst. The dilated fourth ventricle is below the level of the cerebellar vermis.

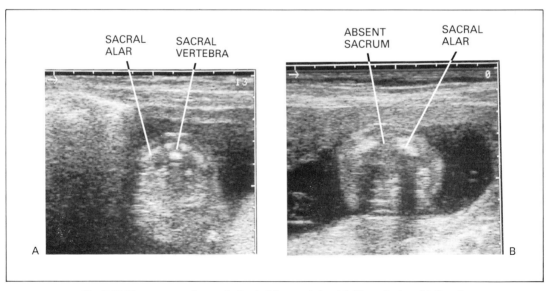

Fig. 7.18 Transverse sections at the level of the sacral alar. (a) Normal spine. (b) Sacral agenesis.

who have insulin dependent diabetes mellitus. It ranges in severity from absence of the sacrum with short femora to complete fusion of the lower limbs — the mermaid syndrome (sirenomelia). Figure 7.18a demonstrates the normal sacrum seen in cross-section at the level of the sacral alar. Figure 7.18b clearly demonstrates absence of the sacrum.

CHAPTER EIGHT
Other fetal anomalies

GASTROINTESTINAL DISORDERS

These conditions usually present because of a raised MSAFP, polyhydramnios, or abnormal ultrasound findings on routine examination for establishing gestational age.

Bowel obstruction

Amniotic fluid is usually removed by fetal swallowing and subsequent absorption by the fetal bowel. In cases of bowel obstruction, absorption is decreased and polyhydramnios occurs. Bowel that is proximal to the obstruction becomes filled with fluid and is, therefore, easily recognised.

Duodenal atresia is an easy ultrasound diagnosis to make because of the classic 'double bubble' appearance (Fig. 8.1). Although the lesion is surgically correctable it may be associated with Down syndrome (trisomy 21) so the fetus should be karyotyped. The main differential diagnosis is with the much rarer condition of a *choledochal cyst* (Fig. 8.2). In cases of duodenal atresia it should be possible to make the bubbles join up at the pylorus. The stomach bubble is usually equal in size or larger than the duodenal bubble. Choledochal cysts are often bigger than the stomach bubble, do not connect with the stomach and are not associated with polyhydramnios. They are rarely associated with chromosome abnormalities but should be removed soon after birth as they cause obstructive jaundice. *Jejunal atresia* produces a 'triple bubble' appearance (Fig. 8.3).

Small bowel obstruction may also be due to *meconium ileus*. This condition is associated with cystic fibrosis and on ultrasound the bowel appears hyperechoic. Occasionally the bowel will rupture and free fluid with intraperitoneal calcification may be seen. As the commonest gene that causes cystic fibrosis has now been cloned the parents should be

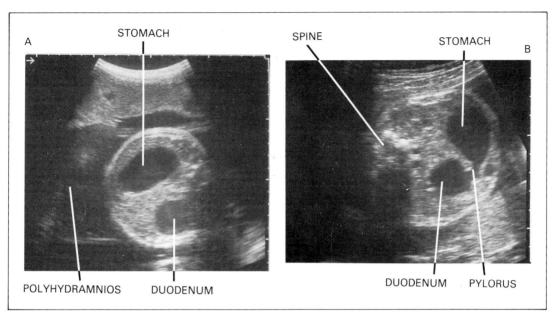

Fig. 8.1 (a) Transverse section of the fetal abdomen demonstrating the double bubble appearance of duodenal atresia. (b) An oblique view demonstrating the connection between the stomach and the duodenum.

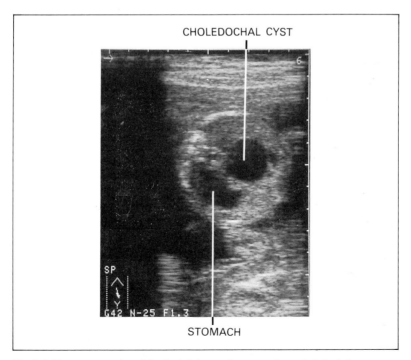

Fig. 8.2 Transverse section of the fetal abdomen demonstrating a choledochal cyst.

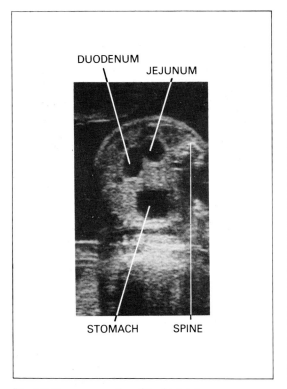

Fig. 8.3 Transverse section of the fetal abdomen demonstrating the triple bubble appearance of jejunal atresia. The patient also has polyhydramnios.

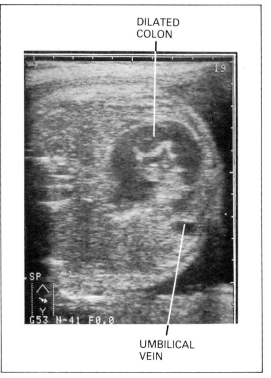

Fig. 8.4 Transverse section of the fetal abdomen at 34 weeks gestation demonstrating a dilated loop of colon due to a volvulus secondary to malrotation of the gut. The diagnosis was made antenatally by the intermittent nature of the obstruction.

tested. Bright echoes from the small bowel may also be due to prenatal hypoxia or virus infection.

Large bowel obstruction is usually only seen in late pregnancy. Care should be taken as normal colon is visible in late pregnancy (Fig. 6.24). Figure 8.4 demonstrates dilated colon due to malrotation and a subsequent *volvulus*, which is probably the commonest cause of late dilatation. It is an intermittent dilatation and may be associated with polyhydramnios. It rarely requires antenatal intervention but if confirmed by postnatal barium studies the child should have the malrotation surgically corrected. Other causes of distended large bowel are rare but include *Hirschsprung's syndrome* (Fig. 8.5). This may be suspected in antenatally diagnosed large bowel obstruction as the rectum is not visualised.

The oesophagus cannot be reliably visualised by ultrasound. Failure to identify a stomach bubble on repeated occasions should raise the possibility of *oesophageal atresia*.

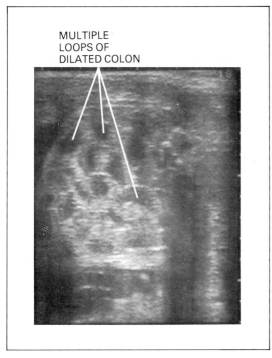

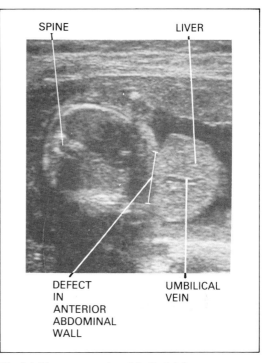

Fig. 8.5 Transverse section of the fetal abdomen at 35 weeks gestation demonstrating multiple dilated loops of bowel. The diagnosis of Hirschsprung's disease was made postnatally.

Fig. 8.6 Transverse section of the fetal abdomen demonstrating an anterior abdominal wall defect of an omphalocoele. Note the umbilical vein is seen outside the abdominal cavity.

Omphalocoele/gastroschisis

Both these conditions may present because of a raised MSAFP. They are defects in the anterior abdominal wall and so should be detectable when the AC is being measured in the routine early scan.

Omphalocoele is a failure of the gut to return to the abdominal cavity after the physiological herniation at 8 weeks gestation. This results in a midline defect in the abdominal wall through which protrudes a peritoneal sac containing liver, small bowel, stomach and perhaps colon. Figure 8.6 illustrates the ultrasound appearances of an omphalocoele. In severe cases the midline defect may extend into the chest such that the fetal heart is outside the body cavity (ectopia cordis) or down into the pelvis so that the bladder is involved (ectopia vesicae).

Most omphalocoeles are surgically repairable after birth; however, up to 50% may be associated with chromosomal or cardiac lesions. Before offering a prognosis, therefore, the fetus should be karyotyped and a detailed cardiac scan should be performed. If the pregnancy continues, vaginal delivery may be considered as the omphalocoele

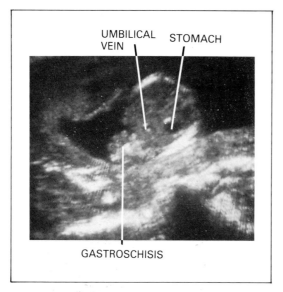

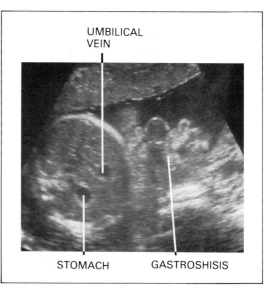

Fig. 8.7 Transverse section of a fetal abdomen at 17 weeks gestation demonstrating the free floating loops of bowel of a gastroschisis.

Fig. 8.8 Transverse section of a fetal abdomen at 29 weeks gestation demonstrating a gastroschisis. Note the normal amount of amniotic fluid.

rarely causes dystocia and the toughened peritoneal sac is rarely ruptured during delivery.

Gastroschisis is a rarer condition in which there is a defect in the umbilical ring. The defect is smaller than that of an omphalocoele and allows only the small bowel to escape into the amniotic cavity. The bowel is not usually covered by peritoneum. The characteristic appearance (Figs 8.7 & 8.8) of free floating bowel makes its differentiation from omphalocoele relatively easy. It is usually an isolated defect, i.e. it is not associated with other anomalies. Surgical repair is easy after birth but bowel resection may be necessary because of stenosis.

Figure 8.9 illustrates an umbilical hernia. The hernia contains only a loop of small bowel which is confined within the umbilical cord. The condition is intermittent and therefore may easily be overlooked on a single examination. There is a small association with chromosome abnormalities (about 1%).

None of the above conditions show any tendency to be recurrent.

CHEST ABNORMALITIES

Diaphragmatic hernia

The defect in the diaphragm is commonly left-sided; stomach, colon and even spleen may enter the fetal chest. The heart is often pushed

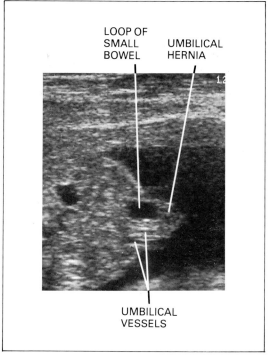

LOOP OF
SMALL   UMBILICAL
BOWEL   HERNIA

UMBILICAL
VESSELS

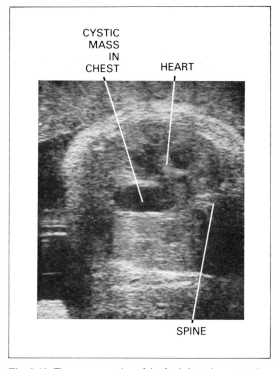

CYSTIC
MASS
IN
CHEST   HEART

SPINE

Fig. 8.9 Oblique section of the fetal abdomen at the level of the cord insertion demonstrating an umbilical hernia. Note that this is a herniation of the small bowel into the umbilical cord. The fetus was an example of trisomy 13.

Fig. 8.10 Transverse section of the fetal chest demonstrating a cystic space alongside the fetal heart.

into the right side of the chest, and although it is usually structurally normal it is often difficult to determine if the major vessels are correctly connected. The diagnosis is suspected by the finding of cystic structures within the chest (Fig. 8.10) and confirmed by demonstrating a defect in the diaphragm (Fig. 8.11). The defect is usually not directly visualised but is inferred by seeing parts of the bowel passing through the diaphragm (Fig. 8.11).

It is probable that there are times when neither the stomach nor the colon are in the fetal chest so that the diagnosis of diaphragmatic hernia may not be apparent on routine scanning in early pregnancy. A clue, however, is a swan-neck bend in the fetal descending aorta (Fig. 8.12) and if present this should lead to prolonged or repeated examination.

Although the defect in the diaphragm is readily amenable to surgery, up to 50% of neonates will die from associated pulmonary hypoplasia. Lung size cannot easily be assessed by ultrasound but the babies that will die demonstrate left ventricular compression as early as 22–24 weeks gestation. The left ventricular size is easily measured by means of M-mode and should be almost the same as the right ventricle.

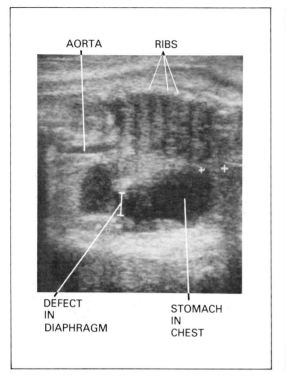

Fig. 8.11 Longitudinal view of the fetus in Figure 8.10 demonstrating an obvious defect in the diaphragm and the stomach in the fetal chest.

Fig. 8.12 The swan-neck bend of the descending aorta suggesting the presence of a diaphragmatic hernia.

Antenatally the pregnancies are usually not complicated although impaired absorption of amniotic fluid by the fetal gut may cause polyhydramnios. If much of the colon is in the fetal chest this may result in a reduced AC measurement, giving the impression of asymmetrical growth retardation. Serial measurements, however, usually demonstrate normal growth velocity.

In the paediatric literature diaphragmatic herniae are usually reported as isolated defects, but evidence of an association with chromosome abnormalities is accumulating from their prenatal diagnosis. The risk is approximately 15% and we currently recommend karyotyping before giving a prognosis.

Cystic adenomatoid malformation

This is a rare malformation which is readily diagnosed on ultrasound but is often confused with diaphragmatic hernia. The lesion is usually unilateral and may be one of three types:

Type I. This type has large cysts (usually more than 10 mm in diameter) and is usually confined to a single lobe.

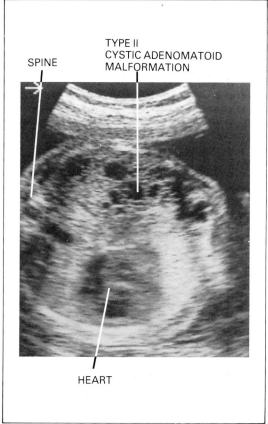

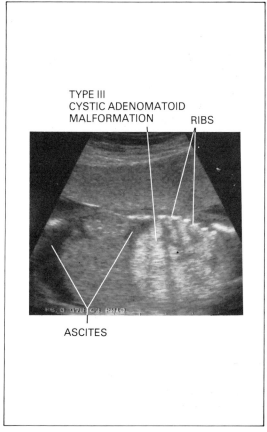

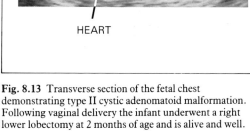

Fig. 8.13 Transverse section of the fetal chest demonstrating type II cystic adenomatoid malformation. Following vaginal delivery the infant underwent a right lower lobectomy at 2 months of age and is alive and well.

Fig. 8.14 Longitudinal section of a fetus demonstrating type III cystic adenomatoid malformation of the lungs together with fetal ascites. The pregnancy was terminated.

Type II. This type has smaller cysts and again may be confined to a single lobe (Fig. 8.13).

Type III. This involves microcysts such that the individual cysts are not resolved on ultrasound examination but the whole lung appears bright (Fig. 8.14).

Types I & II rarely cause antenatal problems and, although a lobectomy is usually required soon after birth to prevent superimposed infections, the longterm prognosis is excellent. Type III has an extremely poor prognosis such that termination should be considered. It may be associated with hydrops fetalis and polyhydramnios in which case there have been no reported survivors.

URINARY TRACT ANOMALIES

The commonest reasons for referral in these cases are oligohydramnios, abnormal ultrasound findings or a previous history of an affected infant.

The method for scanning kidneys and the recommended measurements are to be found in Chapter 6.

After 16 weeks gestation the majority of amniotic fluid is fetal urine. Any decrease in urine production or obstruction of the urinary tract will cause oligohydramnios. In renal agenesis there is always severe oligohydramnios. This, together with the accompanying fetal flexion, makes the diagnosis difficult. Furthermore, only one renal area is usually available for examination as the other lies in the acoustic shadow of the spine. In addition, the renal fat pad or a large adrenal gland may well mimic a renal echo. If the fetal bladder is seen to fill, this effectively excludes the diagnosis of renal agenesis. The other major causes of oligohydramnios are severe growth retardation and ruptured membranes. Unfortunately, fetal bladder filling, even in response to maternally administered frusemide, is usually absent in both renal agenesis and growth retardation. The prognosis in cases of severe oligohydramnios is poor, regardless of the cause. However, unless you are sure of the diagnosis the correct course is probably to err on the side of refuting the diagnosis of renal agenesis and to allow nature to take her course.

Other methods of resolving the cause of oligohydramnios in the second trimester are Doppler ultrasound examination (Ch. 13) and amnio-infusion. The latter involves the instillation of sufficient normal saline (50–500 ml), coloured with a small amount of methylene blue, via an amniocentesis needle to allow appropriate visualisation. This is best performed with monitoring of intra-amniotic pressure as it may result in rupture of the membranes. If the cause of the oligohydramnios is rupture of the membranes, the vaginal discharge will become blue.

Congenital cystic disease of the kidney

Unilateral isolated cysts of the fetal kidney are rare and harmless. All that is necessary prenatally is to ensure that the AC is not so large as to prevent safe vaginal delivery. As isolated renal cysts arise from the substance of the kidney they are easily distinguished from pelvi-ureteric junction obstruction which is the main differential diagnosis.

Infantile polycystic kidney disease is a lethal condition which has an autosomal recessive inheritance pattern. This means that there is a one in four chance of recurrence. The disease is diagnosable prenatally but not always with ease. The condition is always bilateral, with cysts that may vary in size from microscopic to several millimetres. The size of the cysts determines the ultrasound appearance. Microcysts tend to be

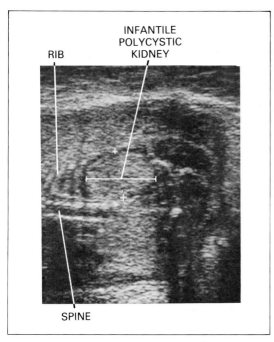

RIB

INFANTILE
POLYCYSTIC
KIDNEY

SPINE

Fig. 8.15 Longitudinal view of a fetus with infantile polycystic kidneys. Microscopic kidney cysts make the kidney much more echogenic than the fetal lungs. Compare the echogenicity of this kidney with the normal kidney demonstrated in Figure 6.28.

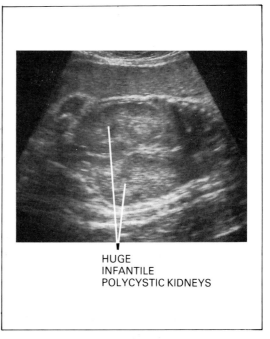

HUGE
INFANTILE
POLYCYSTIC KIDNEYS

Fig. 8.16 Longitudinal section of a fetus at 32 weeks demonstrating large, bright polycystic kidneys. Note the oligohydramnios.

found in normal-sized kidneys and produce only an increase in echogenicity (Fig. 8.15). Kidneys containing microcysts tend to grow throughout pregnancy (Fig. 8.16), so we recommend serial examinations in women who are at increased risk.

Multicystic kidneys are kidneys that demonstrate large cysts (Figs 8.17 & 8.18) with little or no remaining renal tissues. They are thought to be the end result of obstruction to the ureter or bladder. If the condition is unilateral, and the contralateral kidney is normal, a good prognosis can be made. Antenatally, having made the diagnosis, all that is necessary is to monitor the AC to ensure that a safe vaginal delivery will be possible. Nephrectomy may be necessary after birth as the kidney tends to be a source of recurrent infection and/or hypertension. Bilateral multicystic kidney disease is always associated with severe oligohydramnios and has a poor outlook. The finding of large cysts in the fetal kidney with a normal amount of amniotic fluid should raise the possibility of the antenatal expression of adult polycystic kidney disease. This is an autosomal dominant condition and so both parents should have their kidneys scanned. Adult polycystic kidney disease tends not to produce symptoms until the fifth decade of life.

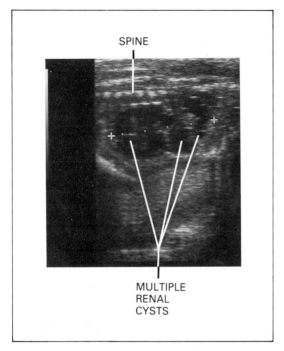

Fig. 8.17 Longitudinal section of a multicystic kidney at 30 weeks gestation. The cysts could not be made to join the renal pelvis.

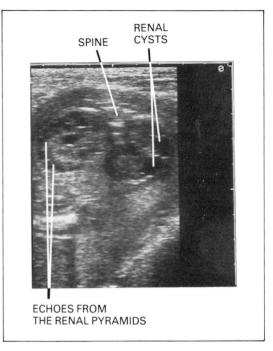

Fig. 8.18 Transverse section of the fetal kidneys from the patient illustrated in Figure 8.17. Note that the peripherally distributed echo free areas seen in the right kidney are a normal appearance in late pregnancy and are due to urine within the renal pyramids.

Obstructive uropathy

This is the name given to a range of conditions in which there is an obstruction at some point in the urinary tract. They are usually detected because of oligohydramnios or abnormal ultrasound findings.

In the worst form (*urethral stenosis or atresia*) there is very severe oligohydramnios and bilateral dysplastic kidneys (see below). The fetus is invariably male and usually dies in utero. The condition can usually be distinguished from renal agenesis or early severe intrauterine growth retardation by the dilatation of the urinary tract (Fig. 8.19).

The most favourable form of obstructive uropathy is *pelvi-ureteric junction obstruction* (PUJO). The appearances are illustrated in Figure 8.20. There is always a dilated renal pelvis which commonly has an extrarenal extension. Usually, however, the renal cortex is well preserved and renal function remains excellent. There are always adequate amounts of amniotic fluid and the fetal bladder can be observed to fill and empty. Hourly fetal urinary production rates (HFUPR) are normal. PUJO is usually caused by a neuromuscular

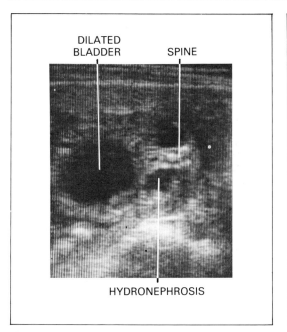

Fig. 8.19 Transverse section of the fetal abdomen demonstrating a grossly dilated bladder.

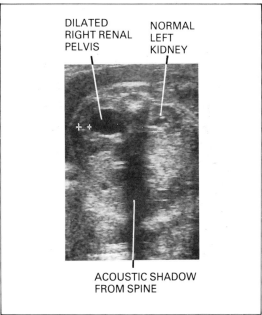

Fig. 8.20 Transverse section demonstrating right-sided pelvi-ureteric junction obstruction (PUJO). The cursors illustrate measurement of the maximum, renal cortex which was normal at 8 mm.

defect at the junction of the ureter and the renal pelvis but occasionally may be caused by an aberrant renal artery. It is often bilateral although it may be expressed unilaterally in utero. We recommend monthly monitoring of maximum renal cortical thickness. Figure 8.21 illustrates two cases. Case (a) demonstrates the usual finding of little or no decline in cortical thickness and consequently a good outcome. Case (b) and Figure 8.22 demonstrate the much rarer progressive deterioration resulting in a nonfunctioning kidney that was later removed. If there is obvious deterioration in the thickness of the renal cortex, preterm delivery should be considered.

After delivery the infant should be reviewed regularly by a paediatric urologist. Most commonly the condition does not worsen, but surgery, in the form of a pyeloplasty, may be necessary because of repeated urinary tract infections. Large, nonfunctioning kidneys may shrivel after birth but if not they are best removed as they are the source of recurrent infections and of hypertension in later life.

Most operators recognise PUJO by its obvious appearance but this may be difficult in borderline cases. We suggest that if the mean of the transverse and anteroposterior diameters of the renal pelvis is greater than 8 mm this should warrant both antenatal and paediatric follow-up.

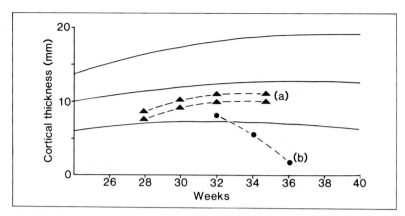

Fig. 8.21 Charts of maximum cortical thickness illustrating two cases of PUJO. (a) The cortical thickness remains within normal limits throughout the pregnancy. This is the usual course for PUJO. (b) Deteriorating cortical thickness. This kidney did not function after birth and was later removed.

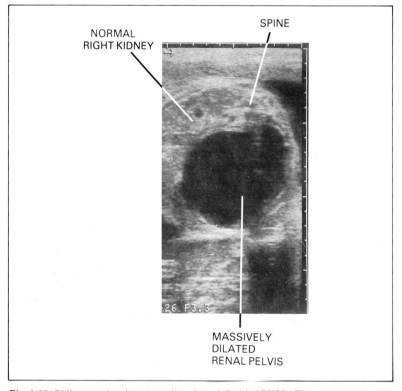

Fig. 8.22 Oblique section demonstrating a huge left-sided PUJO. The cortex was so thin that it could not be measured. The right kidney was normal and there was a normal amount of amniotic fluid. Following delivery the kidney did not function and was later removed.

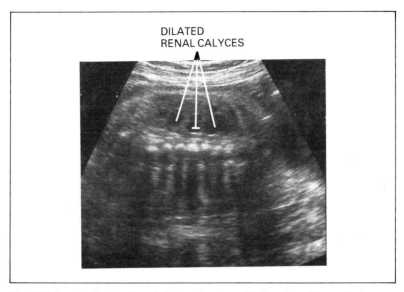

Fig. 8.23 Longitudinal section of a kidney showing mild dilatation of the renal calyces. The echo free spaces were not renal cysts as continuity could be demonstrated with the renal pelvis.

It is worth remembering that the obstruction is intermittent and may vary in severity from one examination to the next. For this reason, all cases of PUJO diagnosed antenatally should have a minimum of two ultrasound examinations postnatally (usually performed at 3 days and 3 months of age) before the condition can be confidently excluded.

Most cases of PUJO are not associated with chromosomal abnormalities. In the absence of other structural markers (Appendix 3) we suggest that karyotyping should only be performed for severe obstruction of early onset or in cases of associated ureteric dilatation suggesting ureteric reflux.

The diagnosis of PUJO depends upon finding a dilated renal pelvis but there may also be dilatation of the renal calyces (Fig. 8.23). In longitudinal section these may be mistaken for a multicystic kidney but in PUJO the dilated renal pelvis can be made to join the calyces.

Between these two extreme groups (urethral stenosis/atresia and PUJO) there is a group in which prognosis is difficult. The fetus is usually male and presents with mild to moderate oligohydramnios and some degree of dilatation of the urinary tract. The commonest cause of this condition is *posterior urethral valves*. These are folds of mucosa at the bladder neck that act as a one-way valve and prevent urine from leaving the bladder. As they are present from early in fetal life they cause problems from the time that the fetal kidneys start to produce urine. They cause back pressure which affects the development of the kidneys. The kidneys invariably show some degree of dysplasia, the degree depending upon how completely the bladder is obstructed. The dysplastic parts of the kidney effectively have no function. Outcome therefore depends upon how much normal kidney remains. It is ultrasonically difficult to determine the degree of dysplasia; if it is visible at all it shows as areas of increased echogenicity within the kidney. Urethral valves may also be associated with other anomalies such as chromosomal anomalies, bowel atresias and cranio-spinal defects.

A few fetuses with severe obstruction due to posterior urethral valves may have their lives saved by vesico-amniotic shunting. This involves insertion of a suprapubic catheter into the fetal bladder under ultrasound control in order to bypass the obstruction caused by the urethral valves. Even with careful selection of fetuses thought to be suitable for such treatment, only about one quarter will survive.

Most forms of obstructive uropathy are sporadic, and recurrence is unlikely. We recommend, however, that a detailed anomaly scan should be offered to these women in their next pregnancy at 16–20 weeks gestation, and that serial scans would be reassuring for both the woman and the clinician.

SKELETAL ABNORMALITIES

Commonly, women are referred because of a past or personal history of a limb reduction deformity, or the limbs are found to be short on routine ultrasound.

The syndromes involving the limbs are bewildering and do not fit into an easy classification. However, for the purposes of ultrasound they may be classified according to how they may be detected, as follows:

- Absence of limbs
  — Complete absence (amelia)
  — Partial absence of a limb or segment of a limb (meromelia)
  — Absence of long bones with the hands and/or feet attached to the body (phocomelia)
- Shortening of the long bones (Fig. 8.24). Many syndromes associated with limb reduction deformities are not apparent before 24 weeks gestation (Table 8.1) and can only be detected by serial fortnightly measurements starting from 16 weeks gestation. Fortunately, those limb reduction deformities that are lethal, usually because of an associated small ribcage, are apparent in early pregnancy (Table 8.2). Figures 8.25–8.27 illustrate a camptomelic dwarf
- Defective mineralisation and/or fracture.

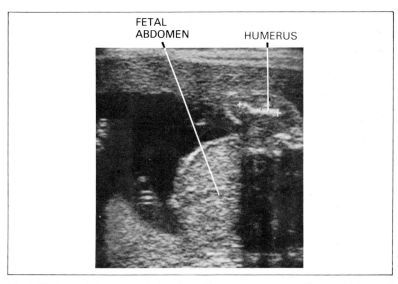

Fig. 8.24 A case of thanotophoric dwarfism. The humerus measures 19 mm which is well below the lower limit for 24 weeks gestation. The fetus also had a small chest and a 'cloverleaf' skull making a definitive prenatal diagnosis possible.

Table 8.1 Less than lethal limb reduction syndromes

Syndrome	Inheritance	Limbs	Other features
Achondroplasia	AD	Late onset micromelia	Megalocephaly Mild hydrocephaly
Hypochondroplasia	AD	Late onset micromelia	
Acromesomelia	AR	Micromelia: distal > proximal	
Ellis van Creveld	AR	Late onset micromelia	Small thorax Polydactyly ASD
Diastrophic dysplasia	AR	Micromelia Hitch-hiker thumbs	
Arthrogryposis	—	Flexion deformities Extended elbow, flexed wrist	Flexion deformities Talipes Oligohydramnios IUGR

AD: Autosomal dominant
AR: Autosomal recessive

It is our practice to only measure the femur in routine cases and in cases referred for anomaly scans for reasons other than skeletal deformities. We check that the other limbs are present and that they appear to be the correct length.

In a woman with a past or personal history of limb deformities, serial detailed scans are often necessary.

Table 8.2 Lethal limb reduction deformities

Syndrome	Inheritance	Limbs	Other features
Achondrogenesis	AR	Severe micromelia	Poorly calcified sacrum Hydrops Polyhydramnios
Thanatophoric	Usually sporadic	Severe micromelia 'Telephone receiver' femurs	Small chest Megalocephaly Cloverleaf skull Absent corpus callosum Polyhydramnios
Jeune's asphyxiating thoracic dystrophy	AR	Severe micromelia	Polydactyly Dysplastic kidneys Small chest
Camptomelic dystrophy	AR	Severe micromelia	Small chest Bowed tibia and femur Macrocephaly VSD Cleft palate Polyhydramnios

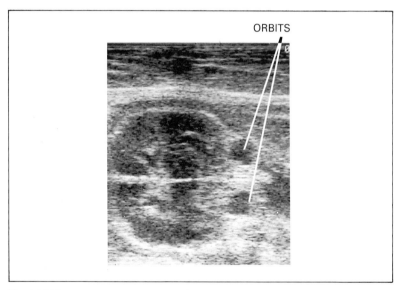

Fig. 8.25 The unusual appearance of the fetal orbits in a case of camptomelic dwarfism. On initial inspection the orbits appeared small and close together, but careful measurement demonstrated macrocephaly with normal orbits.

Morphology and mineralisation (Table 8.3)

The normal femur may appear to be mildly bowed after 18 weeks gestation. Abnormal curvature usually suggests camptomelic dwarfism.

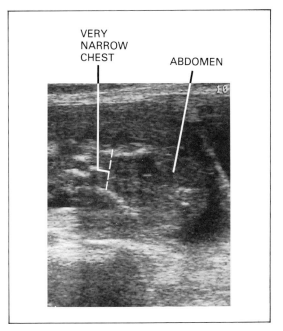

Fig. 8.26 This demonstrates the extremely narrow chest of the fetus illustrated in Figures 8.25 & 8.27.

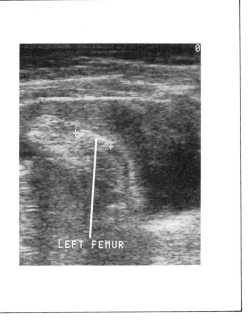

Fig. 8.27 The left femur of the fetus illustrated in the previous two pictures. The femur measured 9 mm which was well outside the normal range for 26 weeks gestation.

Table 8.3 Syndromes of decreased mineralisation

Syndrome	Inheritance	Ultrasonic features
Hypophosphatasia	AR	Homozygous — decreased mineralisation, bowed tibia Heterozygous — probably not detectable
Hypophosphatasia	X-linked	Not detectable
Osteogenesis imperfecta (type I)	AD	Micromelia after midpregnancy Bowed limbs Syndactyly Umbilical hernia
Osteogenesis imperfecta (type II)	AR	Severe early micromelia Intrauterine fractures Hydrocephaly

The degree of mineralisation of the bones is difficult to assess. In osteogenesis imperfecta congenita, however, the demineralisation is usually severe and may be associated with fractures of the long bones and ribs. In achondrogenesis the spine is often severely demineralised and this can be visualised ultrasonically.

Hands and feet

These are commonly involved in syndromes of abnormalities. They may be specifically sought because they are the structural markers of more serious underlying abnormalities. The diagnosis is always time consuming and becomes impossible if there is oligohydramnios. The most common abnormalities are:

- Club foot (1 per 1000 live births). This is diagnosed when the whole length of the foot can be seen in the same section as the tibia and fibula (Fig. 8.28). This is often a marker of more serious conditions but will almost inevitably occur with marked oligohydramnios
- Absent digits
- Extra digits — polydactyly (Fig. 8.29)
- Fused digits — syndactyly and ectrodactyly
- Clinodactyly. This is marked curving of any finger, but is most common in the little finger. It is usually due to hypoplasia of the middle phalanx.

Scanning the hand is made difficult because the fetus commonly has its hands closed into tight fists. However, if it is necessary to examine the hands then the extended fingers and the metacarpal bones should be demonstrated as this excludes fusion defects.

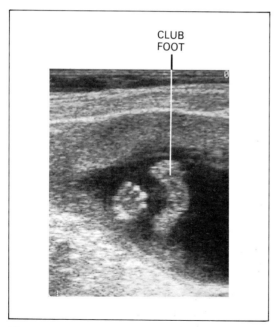

Fig. 8.28 A normal fetal hand and a club foot. There were no other abnormalities present and the karyotype was normal.

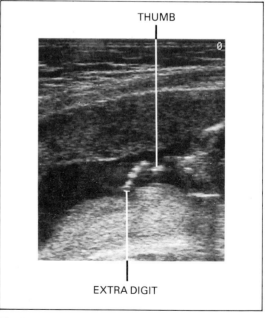

Fig. 8.29 An example of polydactyly. As the extra digit is on the ulnar side it is known as postaxial polydactyly.

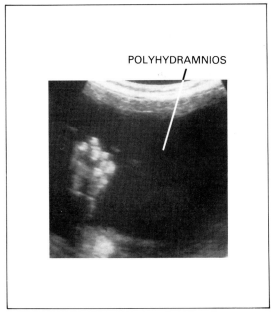

POLYHYDRAMNIOS

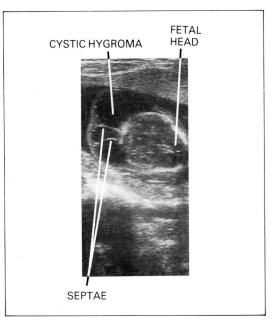

CYSTIC HYGROMA   FETAL HEAD

SEPTAE

Fig. 8.30 A fetal hand at 18 weeks gestation demonstrating overlapping of the second and fifth finger. The fetus was an example of trisomy 18. Note also the polyhydramnios.

Fig. 8.31 Transverse section of the fetal skull illustrating a cystic hygroma. There were no other structural defects but the fetus was an example of Turner's syndrome (45XO).

Figure 8.30 demonstrates the unusual position of the fingers seen in a fetus with trisomy 18.

FETAL TUMOURS

These are very rare but are most often detected at routine ultrasound examinations for establishing gestational age. The commonest lesions are cystic hygromata (pterygium coli). These are abnormalities of the lymphatics that result in cystic swellings around the fetal neck. Many of them are associated with Turner's syndrome (45 XO), in which case there is often fetal hydrops. Cystic hygromata should not be confused with encephalocoeles as the latter have a bony defect in the skull. Cystic hygromata also have septa (Fig. 8.31). If cystic hygromata are discovered the fetus should be karyotyped to exclude Turner's syndrome. If the karyotype is normal the pregnancy may be allowed to continue as the hygromata are surgically correctable after birth.

The second most common tumour that may be encountered is a teratoma. These are commonly sacrococcygeal (Fig. 8.32) but may also occur in the fetal neck. They are usually a mixture of solid and cystic structures but the solid components predominate. About a third will

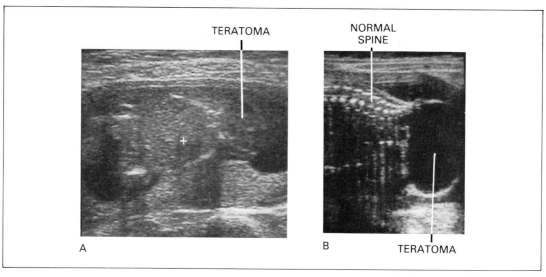

Fig. 8.32 Sacrococcygeal teratoma. (a) Transverse section demonstrating the usual appearance of a solid tumour. (b) A less common example where the teratoma is entirely cystic. This fetus was referred with a diagnosis of spina bifida but the spine was entirely normal.

become malignant with time, but malignancy is rarely present at birth. Caesarean section is usually necessary to deliver the infant because of the size of the tumour. Sacrococcygeal teratomas have a good prognosis although paediatric surgery may be difficult if there is a pelvic extension. Teratomas of the fetal neck (Fig. 8.33) also involve the fetal face and if they extend above the maxilla they are fatal. Teratomas confined to the neck have a 50% operative mortality and delivery has to be by Caesarean section.

UMBILICAL CORD

The umbilical cord should contain two arteries and one vein. Figure 8.34 demonstrates a single umbilical artery. 80% of fetuses with a single artery are normal, but it may be associated with abnormalities of the urinary tract, heart, gastrointestinal system and external ear. If an associated abnormality is found, the fetus should be karyotyped.

GENITALIA

Figure 8.35 demonstrates bilateral hydrocoeles. This finding should prompt a search for intra-abdominal pathology such as ascites or an

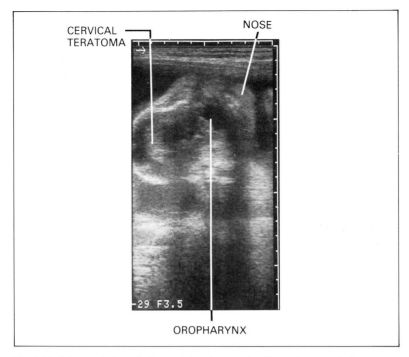

Fig. 8.33 Submental view of a fetus at 34 weeks gestation illustrating a cervical teratoma. The infant was delivered by Caesarean at 38 weeks but died shortly after birth.

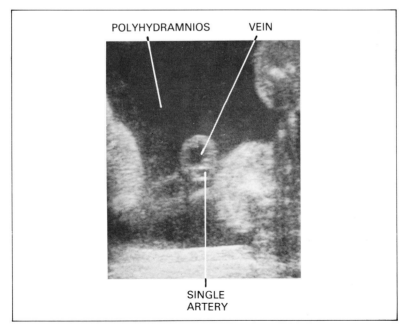

Fig. 8.34 Transverse section of the umbilical cord demonstrating a single artery.

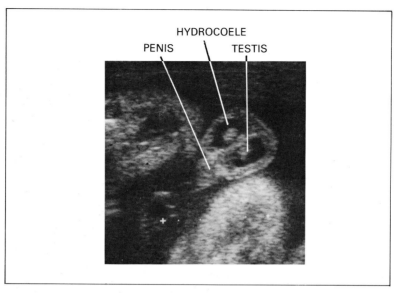

Fig. 8.35 Bilateral hydrocoeles.

intra-abdominal cyst. In the absence of such pathology the patient may be reassured as the hydrocoeles will resolve spontaneously after birth, or are easily surgically correctable.

CARDIAC ANOMALIES

The heart lies in the left side of the chest and occupies approximately one third of the chest cavity. Enlargement of the heart causes the heart to almost fill the chest and the abnormality is therefore usually apparent on simple inspection. Cardiac enlargement may be due to heart failure as part of hydrops fetalis or due to specific abnormalities such as Ebstein's anomaly of downward displacement of the tricuspid valve. The majority of cardiac abnormalities are those in which connections are absent or inappropriate. Connections can be examined using two views based upon views used in paediatric cardiology. These views are the long axis and the short axis view.

Long axis view (four chamber view)

Figure 6.16 illustrates a frozen four chamber view. This view demonstrates the two ventricles, which should appear similar in size, the two atria, the atrioventricular valves and the flap of the foramen ovale. In mitral atresia (hypoplastic left heart) and tricuspid atresia

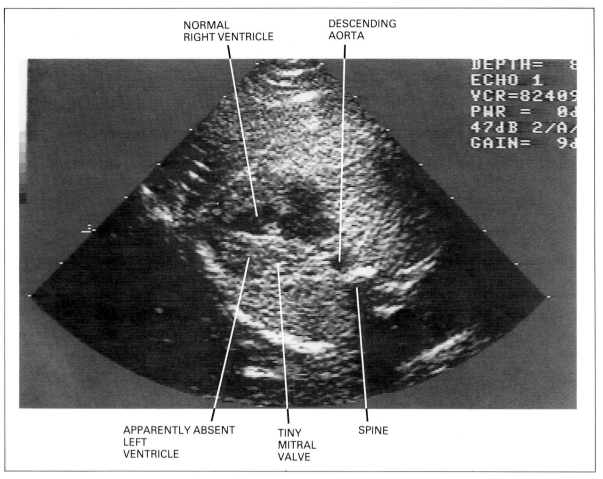

NORMAL
RIGHT VENTRICLE

DESCENDING
AORTA

DEPTH=
ECHO 1
VCR=82409
PWR =   0
47dB 2/A
GAIN=   9

APPARENTLY ABSENT
LEFT
VENTRICLE

TINY
MITRAL
VALVE

SPINE

Fig. 8.36 A 'four chamber view' of a fetal heart demonstrating a hypoplastic left ventricle. A small mitral valve could be visualised but the cavity of the left ventricle was tiny.

(hypoplastic right heart) there is an obvious disparity in size between the two ventricles. In fetal life the right ventricle lies directly beneath the sternum (Fig. 6.16) so it is usually easy to determine which ventricle is small or obliterated. Figure 8.36 demonstrates a case of hypoplastic left heart. Pericardial effusions are easily seen on the four chamber view.

Although the intraventricular septum is seen, it is necessary to demonstrate its continuity with the aorta (Fig. 6.17) in order to exclude a ventricular septal defect. This view is obtained by angling the transducer towards the origin of the aorta. The aorta should then be traced along its course to demonstrate the arch and the descending

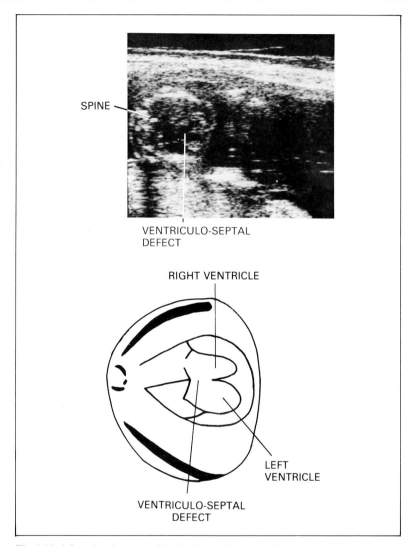

SPINE

VENTRICULO-SEPTAL
DEFECT

RIGHT VENTRICLE

LEFT
VENTRICLE

VENTRICULO-SEPTAL
DEFECT

Fig. 8.37 A four chamber view of the fetal heart demonstrating a ventricularseptal
defect. The fetus also had an overriding aorta with a small pulmonary artery, and was an
example of Fallot's tetralogy.

thoracic aorta. If this proves difficult, then performing the reverse
examination, i.e. finding a longitudinal view of the thoracic aorta and
tracing it to the heart, is often easier. Figure 8.37 demonstrates a
ventricular septal defect.

In order to view the pulmonary trunk, you return to the four
chamber view and angle the transducer in the opposite direction. The
pulmonary trunk appears to leave the right ventricle and travel straight
back towards the fetal spine.

Having completed the above examination most of the common anomalies would be excluded.

Short axis view

This view illustrates the two ventricles and the pulmonary outflow tract. It is the view on which ventricle size is measured.

More detailed examination of the fetal heart involves use of the T–M mode to study rhythm and to determine cavity and ventricular wall measurements — interested readers are referred to a Manual of Fetal Echocardiography (see Further Reading).

Giving a prognosis for most fetal cardiac conditions is difficult because of recent major improvements in cardiac surgery. The parents should therefore be counselled only after discussion with paediatric cardiologists and surgeons.

HYDROPS FETALIS

This is a condition in which there is either fetal ascites, or ascites, pleural and pericardial effusions together with skin oedema. Some of the causes are listed in Table 8.4.

Hydrops was most commonly due to Rhesus isoimmunisation but as Rhesus disease is now rare it is more commonly of the type known as 'non-immune hydrops fetalis'. It is very easily recognised (Fig. 8.38).

Table 8.4 Causes of hydrops fetalis

Classification	Examples
Haematological	Rhesus isoimmunisation
	Twin-twin transfusion
	α-thalassaemia
	Fetal anaemia
Cardiovascular	Paroxysmal dysrhythmias
	Hypoplastic left heart
	Premature closure of foramen ovale
Gastrointestinal	Cirrhosis & portal hypertension
	Hepatitis
	Meconium peritonitis
	Spontaneous bowel perforation
	Bowel stenosis/atresia
Genitourinary	Bladder rupture due to urethral stenosis
Skeletal	Sacrococcygeal teratoma
	Osteogenesis imperfecta
	Asphyxiating thoracic dystrophy
Placental	Angioma
Chromosomal	Down syndrome
	Triploidy
Infective	Cytomegalovirus

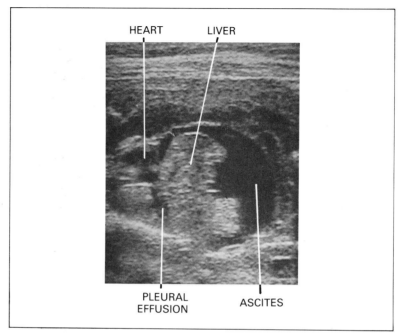

Fig. 8.38 Longitudinal section of a fetus with hydrops fetalis.

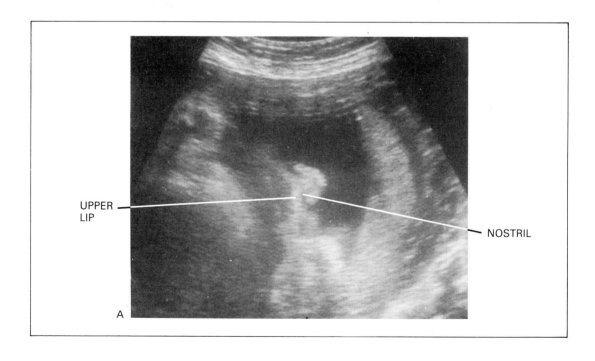

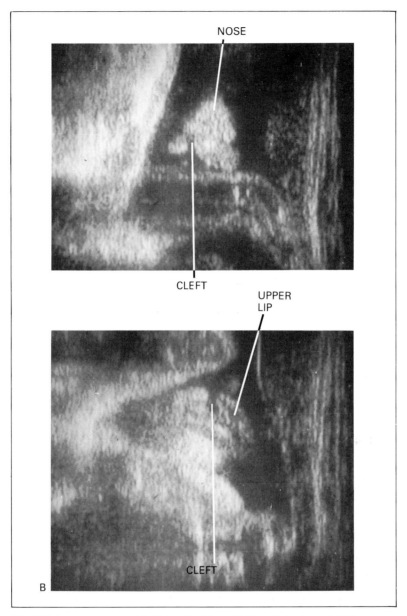

Fig. 8.39 Submental views. (a) Normal fetal lips. (b) Hare lip (unilateral cleft).

In most cases it is fatal either because of the underlying cause or because of pulmonary hypoplasia due to the presence of large pleural effusions. It will rarely resolve without therapy.

Having carefully excluded a structural abnormality it is usually necessary to exclude a chromosomal or infective cause by performing a fetal blood sample. Paroxysmal cardiac dysrhythmias often may only be detected by prolonged (more than 12 hours) fetal heart rate monitoring.

FACIAL ABNORMALITIES

Hare lip and cleft palate are relatively common, occurring in about 1 in 700 pregnancies. Approximately half of such babies will have both abnormalities whilst the remainder will have either one or the other. An isolated cleft palate is a difficult diagnosis but, using the view illustrated in Figure 8.39a, the lips can usually be adequately visualised from 20 weeks onwards. Figure 8.39b illustrates a hare lip.

Abnormalities of the nose and chin are best appreciated from the fetal profile. Figure 8.40 illustrates the very abnormal nose of a fetus with cyclops. Figure 8.41a shows a normal face in profile whilst Figure 8.41b demonstrates micrognathia.

Although hair lip and/or cleft palate commonly occur as single anomalies they may be markers of syndromes. All other facial abnormalities are very commonly associated with syndromes and if

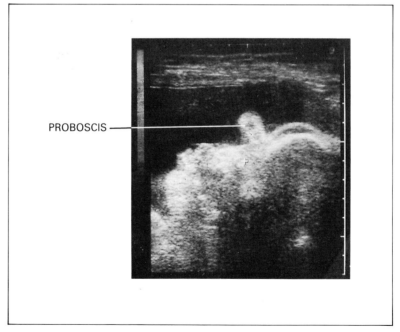

PROBOSCIS

Fig. 8.40 A fetal face in profile at 35 weeks showing a proboscis. This fetus also had cyclops and was an example of the arrhinencephaly–cyclops sequence.

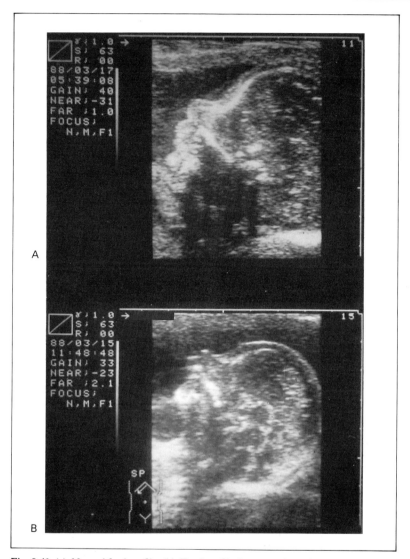

Fig. 8.41 (a) Normal fetal profile. (b) Fetal profile demonstrating micrognathia.

termination is not decided upon on the basis of the ultrasound appearance alone the fetus must be karyotyped.

NUCHAL FAT PAD

This is a recently described structural marker that may suggest the presence of Down syndrome (see also Appendix 3).

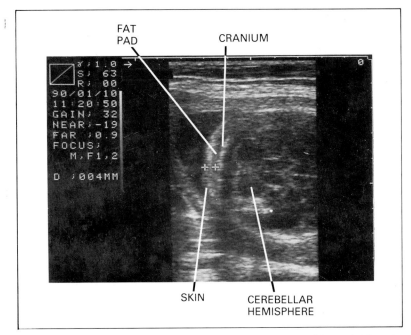

Fig. 8.42 Suboccipitobregmatic view demonstrating measurement of the nuchal fat pad. This was 4 mm (within normal limits).

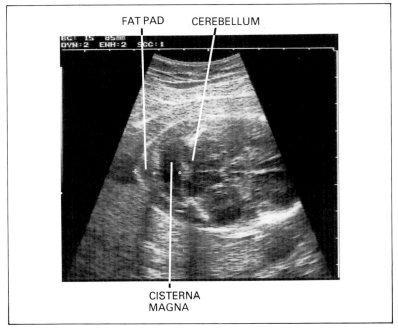

Fig. 8.43 Suboccipitobregmatic view demonstrating a nuchal fat pad in a case of Down syndrome. The pad measures 7.8 mm.

Obtain a suboccipitobregmatic view as used for examining the cerebellum (Fig. 6.6). Measure the fat from the outer table of the occiput to the outer border of the skin. Figure 8.42 demonstrates a normal fat pad whilst that in Figure 8.43 demonstrates a fat pad seen in a fetus with Down syndrome. Care must be taken to measure the fat pad on the views illustrated in Figures 8.42 and 8.43, as measurements taken lower in the fetal neck are dependent upon whether the fetal neck is flexed. Normal fat pads should measure less than 5 mm.

CHAPTER NINE
Invasive procedures performed under ultrasound guidance

AMNIOCENTESIS

Amniocentesis means the removal of amniotic fluid. The indications for its use in both early and late pregnancy are given in Table 9.1.

The involvement of the ultrasonographer with amniocentesis will depend upon how the amniocentesis is carried out. This may be in one of three ways:

1. *With direct ultrasound control.* This means that the person

Table 9.1 Indications for amniocentesis

Early pregnancy
1. For genetic reasons
   a. Maternal age (see Table 9.2)
   b. Previous history of chromosomal anomaly
   c. Balanced translocation in either parent
   d. To determine fetal sex if history of sex-linked disorders
   e. If fetal cardiac lesion, omphalocoele or obstructive uropathy
   f. A history of three or more first trimester abortions
   g. After a triple test★
   h. The presence of structural markers (Appendix 3)
2. For inherited disorders of metabolism
   a. Previous or family history
   b. Racial group
3. Raised MSAFP (high resolution ultrasound is preferable)

Late pregnancy
1. To investigate the extent of Rhesus isoimmunisation
2. To determine fetal lung maturity by lecithin: sphingomyelin ratio (and phosphatidylglycerol)

★ This test is available to some hospitals and is commercially available from St. Bartholomew's hospital. It involves measurement of serum AFP, HCG and plasma oestriols at 15–19 weeks gestation. The results, together with maternal age, are interpreted by a computer programme in order to give a new risk figure for that individual. It is important to note that the test does not exclude the presence of a chromosome abnormality but merely gives a risk figure which may be higher or lower than that based upon maternal age alone.

performing the amniocentesis also performs the preliminary scan to locate the most ideal spot and inserts the needle under direct ultrasound visualisation.

2. *With indirect ultrasound control.* This usually means that the patient is sent for a preliminary ultrasound examination and that the skin is marked to indicate the suggested site of puncture.

3. *Blind, i.e. without ultrasound control.*

We feel strongly that direct ultrasound control should always be used, as it reduces the number of bloody taps and also decreases the risk of injury to both the fetus and the placenta.

Equipment

The following equipment is needed:

- An 18 gauge needle (we find that the 18 gauge Medicut, with the cannula removed, is excellent)
- Two 20 ml syringes
- A sterile dish holding 15–20 ml of 0.5% w/v chlorhexidine in spirit
- Two cotton wool balls
- Two sterile specimen jars of 20–25 ml capacity.

AMNIOCENTESIS IN EARLY PREGNANCY

The most common reason for amniocentesis in early pregnancy is to determine the fetal karyotype. Table 9.2 indicates the maternal age-specific risks of all chromosomal abnormalities. Most area health authorities offer genetic amniocentesis to mothers of 35 years or over.

Amniocentesis is usually performed at about 16 weeks gestation, with the result being available about 3 weeks later. Recently, because of

Table 9.2 Maternal age-specific risks of all chromosome anomalies. (From Ferguson–Smith MA and Yates JRW (1984) Prenatal Diagnosis 4: 5–44, with kind permission of the editor, authors and publishers)

Age (years)	Incidence	Percentage risk
35	1 in 250	0.4
36	1 in 143	0.7
37	1 in 125	0.8
38	1 in 111	0.9
39	1 in 83	1.2
40	1 in 71	1.4
41	1 in 63	1.6
42	1 in 30	3.3
43	1 in 43	2.3
44	1 in 22	4.6
45	1 in 12	8.2

improvements in cell culture techniques, it has become possible to perform amniocentesis for genetic reasons from 10 weeks onwards.

All women should have a preliminary anomaly scan. Amniocentesis will only detect structural anomalies if there is a 'leak' of alphafetoprotein (see Table 7.1). If a structural anomaly is diagnosed on the preliminary scan then the woman may opt for a termination. Serious thought should be given to proceeding with the amniocentesis in such cases, because the structural abnormality may represent a chromosomal problem and karyotyping post-abortal fetal tissue often fails.

Method

A pool of amniotic fluid should be located away from the fetus and the placenta. An anterior placenta rarely covers the entire anterior uterine wall and there is often a 'window' available for a lateral approach. If no window is found then the needle may be put through the anterior placenta, but aiming to avoid the placental edge and the site of the cord insertion.

Direct ultrasound control

Having located a pool of amniotic fluid away from the fetus, the ultrasound transducer is moved slightly away from the spot, but angled to keep the pool in view. The skin over the spot is cleansed with chlorhexidine and the needle is introduced rapidly through the woman's skin and rectus sheath, directed towards the pool. As the needle enters the uterus it is visualised on the ultrasound screen and is advanced under direct ultrasound vision until it can be seen entering the pool.

An assistant should then remove the stilette and aspirate 20 ml of amniotic fluid. If you are on your own it is necessary to put the transducer back in its housing to allow you to aspirate the fluid. The technique of holding the transducer in the operator's left hand whilst visualising an advancing needle held in the operator's right hand is used in amniocentesis, cordocentesis and transabdominal chorion villus sampling.

Indirect ultrasound control

Having located a pool of amniotic fluid away from the fetus, the angle of the transducer to the maternal abdomen is noted together with an approximation of the depth of the pool. A mark is then made on the maternal abdomen at the required spot. This may be done by pressing the hub of a needle into the skin or with the operator's finger nail. We prefer the latter method, as putting a finger under the transducer producers a shadow which should lie over the pool of amniotic fluid chosen. It also prevents the appearance of needles until immediately before you are ready to make the tap.

The skin is then cleansed with chlorhexidine on cotton wool. The needle is then quickly introduced through the woman's skin at the site of the mark. As the painful part is now over, the needle can be gradually guided along the required path so that the operator can feel the structures it is passing through. On entry into the amniotic cavity there is usually a marked 'give'. 20 ml of amniotic fluid should then be aspirated for study. Remove the needle.

At the end of the procedure, irrespective of the technique used, we recommend:

1. Check the fetal heart is still beating and demonstrate it to the woman.

2. Divide the amniotic fluid into two specimen pots. Put 15 ml in one pot for cytogenetic studies, and 5 ml in the other for measurement of AFP.

3. Check the maternal blood group — if she is Rhesus negative, give 250 i.u. of anti-D gammaglobulin intramuscularly. Ideally this should be given immediately following the procedure but in order to be effective it must be given within 72 hours.

The woman should be advised to avoid strenuous physical exercise (including picking up other children) for 48 hours.

Note. If there is an anterior wall fibroid it should be avoided, as pushing the needle through it may produce pain.

Problems

We feel that only two attempts should be made to obtain amniotic fluid on any one occasion.

Maternal obesity. This is rarely sufficient to prevent the use of a Medicut or 18 gauge spinal needle. However, if you are concerned that the needle is going to be too short then measure the depth from the skin surface to the centre of the chosen pool on the ultrasound monitor screen. If it is more than 5 cm then use a long spinal needle.

Failure to aspirate fluid. If you feel that the needle has entered the amniotic cavity then rotate the syringe through 180° and aspirate again. If this fails then use the ultrasound transducer to locate the end of the needle. The needle can be located by the acoustic shadow it produces and by the characteristic echo pattern of its tip (Fig. 9.1). If the needle is not in the amniotic pool then withdraw or advance it until the pool is reached.

If the needle appears to be in an amniotic pool, first check this by scanning in two planes at 90° to each other. If you are convinced it is in an amniotic pool and you are still unable to obtain fluid then push about

1 ml normal saline down the needle and look for turbulence. If no bubbles are seen then either the needle is blocked or you have stripped the chorion from the amnion and the needle is between the membranes. If you have used a needle with a stilette then you may clear a blocked needle by reintroducing the stilette. If this fails then withdraw the needle and start afresh.

Aspirating blood. Stop aspirating and look at the fluid carefully to determine if it is pure blood or if it is blood-stained amniotic fluid. If it is pure blood, remove the needle, check the fetal heart and start again. If it is amniotic fluid stained with old blood then remove 20 ml for examination. If it is fresh blood staining then locate the tip of the needle with the transducer and move the needle into a pool of amniotic fluid. Change the syringe and remove 20 ml of fluid. All blood-stained specimens should be sent to the cytogenetics laboratory as soon as possible as red blood cells are highly toxic to desquamated fetal cells.

Failure to obtain amniotic fluid. If you have had two attempts and you have been unable to obtain amniotic fluid you should abandon the procedure. Rescan the woman to check the fetal heart and to ensure that there is no obvious reason (e.g. oligohydramnios) as to why you have failed. You should defer further attempts for several days or a week (to give time for any blood staining to clear).

TWIN AMNIOCENTESIS

The finding of twins prior to amniocentesis poses counselling and technical problems. On ultrasound examination you should try to determine whether the twins are dizygotic. This is most accurately done if you can show that they are different sexes. The findings of two separate placentae and an obvious dividing membrane (Fig. 9.1) strongly suggest dizygosity. If the fetuses are the same sex you cannot exclude monozygosity and thus the risk of chromosomal abnormality is 1.7 times that of the maternal age-specific risk. If the twins are dizygotic the risk of one twin being chromosomally abnormal is derived as in the following example:

Maternal age = 35 years
Age-specific maternal risk = 1 in 250
Risk for the pregnancy = 1/250 + 1/250
$$= 2/250$$
$$= 1/125$$

If the twins are dizygotic there is usually an obvious membrane between the two sacs and with skill it is possible to tap each sac separately (Fig. 9.1). Some workers inject methylene blue into the first sac after aspiration to ensure that the same sac is not tapped twice; we have not found this necessary. In theory it should only be necessary to

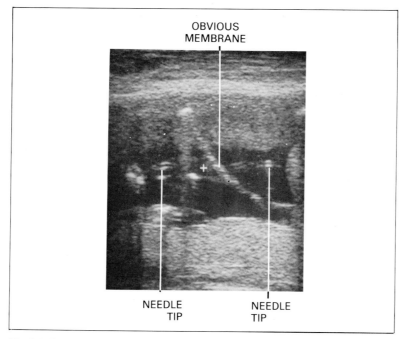

OBVIOUS
MEMBRANE

NEEDLE
TIP

NEEDLE
TIP

Fig. 9.1 Amniocentesis in a dizygotic twin pregnancy. The dividing membrane is clearly seen. There is a needle in each sac, the tips of which are visible as characteristic double echoes.

take one sample from monozygotic twins, but we prefer to take fluid from behind each fetal back as ultrasonically one can never be sure that they are monozygotic twins.

AMNIOCENTESIS IN LATE PREGNANCY

Here the technique is largely the same and you should aim to find a pool of amniotic fluid amongst the fetal limbs as this minimises the risk of damage to a vital fetal part. If this is difficult then attempt to aspirate the pool that can usually be located caudal to the presenting part. Tipping the woman into a head down position often makes this more obvious.

Problems

1. The usual reason for failure to obtain amniotic fluid in late pregnancy is that a lateral approach has been selected and the needle is not long enough. A preliminary measurement of the depth of the amniotic pool will avoid this problem.

2. If the amniocentesis is being performed on a woman with premature rupture of the membranes (PROM),then we find that resting the woman head down for four hours before the procedure usually produces a pool of amniotic fluid that is available to be tapped. This usually means doing the procedure at the woman's bedside.

Note. Do not forget that specimens taken for evaluation of Rhesus disease should be sent to the laboratory in a light-proof container.

Risks

The risks of amniocentesis are indicated in Table 9.3.

Table 9.3 Risks of amniocentesis

Maternal
Damage to bladder, uterus or bowel
Rectus sheath haematoma

Fetal
Damage to a fetal organ
Feto-maternal haemorrhage
Orthopaedic deformities
Increased incidence of respiratory distress syndrome

Overall, there is a 1% risk of fetal death through miscarriage, intrauterine death or preterm delivery.

CORDOCENTESIS

The increasing resolution of the newer ultrasound machines has allowed accurate placement of the needle within the uterus. Under ultrasound guidance fetal skin, liver or kidney may be biopsied but the commonest procedure performed is percutaneous umbilical blood sampling (PUBS), which is also known as cordocentesis. The indications are given in Table 9.4 and the risks are similar to those of amniocentesis (Table 9.3) except that, as it is carried out later in pregnancy (usually 20 weeks or later), the chances of losing a normal pregnancy are probably reduced to the order of 1 in 400. Additional risks of cordocentesis are tamponade or tearing of an umbilical cord vessel.

Equipment

- A sterile dish holding 10–20 ml of 0.5% w/v chlorhexidine in spirit, and two sterile cotton wool balls
- 20 ml of 1% plain lignocaine in a syringe with a 20 gauge needle (blue) attached and a 16 gauge needle (green) to hand

Table 9.4 Indications for cordocentesis

Early pregnancy (20 weeks)
1. Chromosomal analysis
   a. Women who present too late for amniocentesis
   b. Fetuses with a structural abnormality or marker suggestive of a chromosome anomaly (Appendix 3)
2. Viral specific IgM, e.g. toxoplasmosis, rubella, cytomegalovirus
3. Genetic disorders that require fetal blood, e.g. fragile X syndrome, Menke's disease
4. Assessment and treatment of Rhesus disease
5. Exclusion of fetal haemoglobinopathies, e.g. sickle cell disease and thalassaemias. This can also be performed by chorionic villus sampling

Late pregnancy
1. Karyotyping
   a. Fetuses with a structural abnormality or marker suggestive of a chromosome anomaly (Appendix 3)
   b. Severely growth retarded fetuses
   c. Fetuses with an abnormal fetal circulation but a normal uteroplacental circulation (see Ch. 13)
2. Blood gas analysis — in fetuses with absent end-diastolic frequencies (see Ch. 13)
3. Assessment and treatment of Rhesus disease

- A 15 cm 22 gauge spinal needle with its stilette
- Five 1 ml Louer lock syringes
- A pair of sterile, disposable gloves
- A 5 ml ampoule of normal saline
- Appropriate blood bottles
  — Karyotype: a 10 ml plain bottle (white top) into which you have put at least 5000 i.u. heparin
  — Haematology: paediatric (0.5 ml) bottle containing EDTA (pink top)
  — Urea & electrolytes: a paediatric (0.5 ml) bottle containing lithium heparin (orange top)
  — Serum proteins: a plain bottle (white top)
  — Viral studies: a plain bottle (white top).

It is also usual practice to send 20 ml of amniotic fluid at the same time.

Method

This may be a single operator technique but is best performed by two people, one of whom scans the woman whilst the other performs the needling.

Locate the placenta and the cord insertion. Visualise the cord about 1 cm away from the placenta in both the longitudinal and transverse planes. Mark the maternal skin over this site by pressure with a fingernail. Cleanse the skin with chlorhexidine and then raise a small bleb of lignocaine in the skin using the 20 gauge (blue) needle. Change the needle for the 16 gauge (green) needle and infiltrate the subcutaneous tissues, the rectus sheath and the anterior wall of the uterus, aspirating frequently.

As the 15 cm 20 gauge needle is whippy it needs to be steadied during its insertion by grasping its shaft with the operator's sterile gloved left hand. Once the needle has passed the rectus sheath, however, it can usually be guided by the operator's right hand whilst the left hand holds the ultrasound transducer. The needle is moved forward until it punctures the umbilical cord (Fig. 9.2). The tip of the needle should be visualised within the cord in two scanning planes 90° apart and then the stilette is withdrawn.

A 1 ml syringe is attached and blood is aspirated for the appropriate studies. Firm pressure needs to be applied to the syringe in order to aspirate because of the fine bore of the needle. If it is necessary to know whether the needle is in the umbilical vein or the artery, a small amount of normal saline can be flushed down the needle and the direction of the subsequent turbulence observed. Turbulence that flows in the direction of the placenta indicates that the needle is in the umbilical artery.

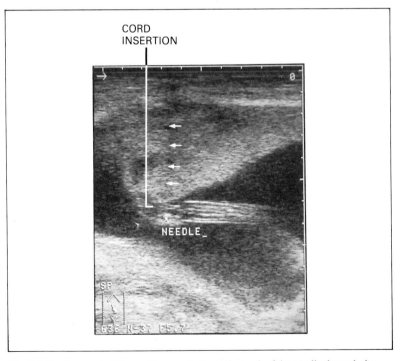

Fig. 9.2 Cordocentesis. The small arrows indicate the track of the needle through the placenta into the cord close to its insertion.

Problems

1. Failure to aspirate blood from the cord. Visualise the tip of the needle in two planes 90° apart — often the needle that appears to be in the cord in one plane has completely missed the cord in the opposite plane. This usually leads to amniotic fluid being aspirated. If the needle appears to be in the cord and blood is not aspirated it suggests that the needle has not entered a cord vessel and it should be advanced or withdrawn until it enters a vessel. If the tip appears to be within a vessel the needle should be flushed with 1 ml of normal saline as fine bore needles commonly block.

2. Fetal bradycardia. A bradycardia as slow as 60 bpm is not uncommon when the cord is first punctured, especially with fetuses under 20 weeks. They usually recover within 60 seconds; if not, the needle should be removed and the procedure repeated at a later date.

3. Unfavourable cord insertion. If the cord insertion into the placenta is not accessible then the intrahepatic portion of the umbilical vein may be used. In this case the needle is directed to pass through the fetal skin and liver. Many operators prefer this approach as the needle is fixed within the baby and is therefore less likely to be dislodged as a result of fetal movement.

The worst situation at cordocentesis is when the cord insertion is into a posteriorly placed placenta and the fetus is facing the placenta. Neither end of the cord is accessible so the choice is either to postpone the procedure or to perform a cardiac stab. If the latter course is felt necessary the tip of the needle is directed through the fetal ribs into one of the ventricles.

CHORION VILLUS SAMPLING

This is usually performed at 9–11 weeks gestation, although it may be carried out transabdominally at any stage in pregnancy. It can be performed transabdominally or transcervically and may be a single operator technique but more commonly involves an operator and another person who performs the ultrasound scan.

Both methods should be preceded by an initial scan performed with an abdominal sector scanner or a vaginal probe to demonstrate fetal viability, gestational age (by crown–rump length measurement), placental site and to determine the presence of any other abnormalities such as fibroids.

The risk of chorion villus sampling is quoted as a 4% chance of losing a normal pregnancy following the procedure. At 9–11 weeks approximately 2% of women will lose a pregnancy after a viable fetus has been seen on ultrasound and therefore the *increased* risk is of the order of 2%. The major advantage of chorion villus sampling is that the results are known sufficiently early in the pregnancy to allow a vaginal termination if an adverse result is obtained.

Currently, chorion villus sampling is not recommended in twin pregnancy, as you cannot guarantee that you have sampled both placentae.

Transcervical approach

Requirements

- 20 ml of 2% aqueous chlorhexidine in a sterile galley pot
- Five sterile gauze squares and a sponge-holding forceps
- An appropriate sized sterile Cusco's speculum
- A sterile tenaculum
- An aspiration cannula. This is a plastic cannula, usually less than 2 mm thick, that contains a malleable aluminium introducer that can be bent to conform to the shape of the uterus
- 20 ml of culture medium containing 4 ml of heparin (5000 units/ml) in a sterile container
- Three 20 ml syringes
- A sterile Petri dish
- A person skilled in recognising chorionic villi that contain blood vessels, and a microscope.

Method

Ideally, the woman should be positioned on a gynaecological examination couch with her legs in low stirrups, but she must be in the lithotomy position with her legs supported. The vulva and vagina are cleansed with aqueous chlorhexidine and a sterile Cusco's speculum is then passed by the operator such that the cervix is visualised. In most cases, the cervix does not need to be grasped with a tenaculum but if it is high in the vagina this may be necessary. After warning the woman that she may experience some low abdominal pain the cervix is grasped and gentle traction applied. In either case, the cervix is then cleansed with aqueous chlorhexidine and dried.

The position of the uterus (anteverted, axial or retroverted) is then determined by ultrasound and the aspiration cannula is bent into the required shape. Under ultrasound guidance the cannula is passed through the cervix and directed into the placental site such that it lies directly beneath the cord insertion (Fig. 9.3). Suction is then applied by means of a 20 ml syringe that contains about 5 ml of culture medium and 1 ml of heparin. Whilst maintaining the suction the needle is then moved to and fro so as to shear off some of the trophoblastic villi. The needle is then removed and the entire contents of the syringe and needle are squirted into a Petri dish. The sample is examined under the

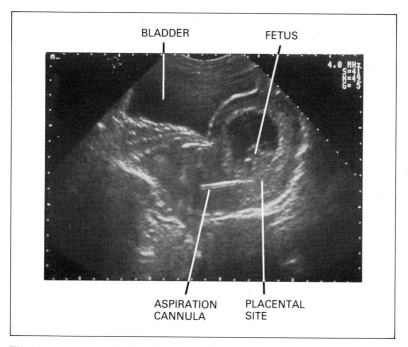

BLADDER   FETUS

4.0 MHZ
S=4
N=4
G=5

ASPIRATION   PLACENTAL
CANNULA   SITE

Fig. 9.3 Transcervical chorion villus sample. The sampling cannula can be seen entering the posteriorly placed placenta.

microscope and should contain villi with visible blood vessels. If these are not present the procedure is repeated.

Single operator techniques require the use of a suction catheter attached to a suction apparatus and the use of a tissue trap. The operator inserts the cannula through the cervix whilst holding the ultrasound transducer in his other hand. The introducer is then withdrawn and the cannula is attached to the suction apparatus. When the cannula is in the correct position occlusion of the hole on the suction tubing allows a continuous negative pressure of 400–500 mmHg to be applied whilst moving the cannula to and fro as above.

Following the procedure the fetal heart is checked and the woman is advised to avoid physical exertion or sexual intercourse for the next 72 hours. If she is Rhesus negative, 250 i.u. of anti-D gammaglobulin should be given intramuscularly.

Problems

1. The presence of vaginal infection. If the vagina is thought to be infected when the speculum is introduced, high vaginal swabs should be taken and the procedure abandoned. The choices are then to perform a transabdominal chorion villus sample or to treat the infection and repeat the procedure at a later date.

2. Inability to obtain sufficient villus material. Ideally some 20–40 mg
of tissue can be obtained and it should contain visible blood vessels, as
this improves the chances of successful culture. If this is not obtained
the technique may be repeated a further two times. If insufficient
material is still not obtained then the procedure should be abandoned
after checking the fetal heart. It may be repeated one week later.

Transabdominal approach

The technique for this approach is similar to that involved in
amniocentesis or cordocentesis. A good sector scanner is required to
demonstrate the pelvic organs. At 8–12 weeks gestation the uterus
tends to be anteverted or retroverted and so presents the placental site
as upper or lower to the abdominal operator (Fig. 9.4). Most workers
use a double needle technique.

Requirements

- 20 ml of 2% aqueous chlorhexidine in a sterile galley pot
- Five sterile gauze squares and a sponge-holding forceps
- An 18 gauge spinal needle and a 20 gauge spinal needle
- 20 ml of culture medium containing 4 ml of heparin (5000 units/ml)
  in a sterile container
- Three 20 ml syringes
- A sterile Petri dish

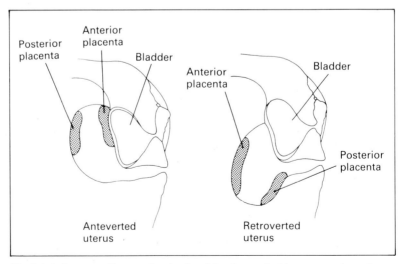

Fig. 9.4 A diagram to illustrate that the site of the placenta is either upper or lower in
early pregnancy. This allows transabdominal chorion villus sampling regardless of
whether the uterus is anteverted or retroverted.

- A person skilled in recognising chorionic villi that contain blood vessels, and a microscope.

Method

Scan the uterus to determine the placental site. Cleanse the skin of the abdomen with the aqueous chlorhexidine. Insert the 18 gauge needle as far as the edge of the placenta. This can usually be done without local anaesthetic, but, for anxious women or operators, the proposed track may be infiltrated with 10 ml of 1% plain lignocaine. Aim for a site towards the centre of the placenta, preferably directly beneath the cord insertion. The placental edge should be avoided as the villi from this site may be hydropic and degenerative and hence may not culture. Remove the stilette and pass the 20 gauge needle down into the placental substance.

Remove the stilette from the 20 gauge needle and attach the 20 ml syringe. Draw the plunger back as far as is comfortably possible in order to create some negative pressure, and then gently move the needle to and fro within the placenta two or three times. Whilst maintaining the negative pressure, withdraw the needle and squirt the contents of the syringe into a Petri dish containing culture medium. Flush the syringe out with the culture medium. The contents of the Petri dish are then examined under the microscope in order to determine if sufficient villi have been obtained. If not, the 20 gauge needle can be reintroduced through the 18 gauge needle, which should be left in position until an adequate sample has been obtained.

Check the fetal heart and demonstrate it to the woman. If the woman is Rhesus negative she should be given 250 i.u. anti-D gammaglobulin intramuscularly.

INDICATIONS FOR CHORION VILLUS SAMPLING

Chromosome analysis

The indications are identical to the genetic reasons given in Table 9.1. Chromosome analysis from chorionic villi may be by direct preparation or by villus culture. Direct preparation gives a result within two days. However, as direct preparations produce less mitoses than culture, the technique is less accurate for detecting minor chromosomal changes and is therefore usually backed up by villus culture.

Results from villus culture are usually available in 7–10 days. Contamination from decidual cells may lead to an overgrowth of maternal cells and hence give a false result. This does not happen with the direct preparation, so ideally both techniques should be employed.

Finally, as the tissue being tested for chromosomes comes from the placenta (trophoblast) it may not demonstrate the same karyotype as the fetus in about 2% of cases. In most of these cases, this results in a trisomy 2, 16 or 20 being reported and although these would be lethal to the fetus they do not appear to affect the placenta. In such cases an amniocentesis should be performed in later pregnancy to determine the fetal karyotype.

DNA analysis

As placental tissue is actively growing, it is rich in DNA and chorionic villi can therefore be used for gene probing. This may be performed by a direct gene probe or by a more complex method involving restriction fragment length polymorphisms (RFLPs).

Once the gene associated with a condition has been cloned, a radioactive probe can be prepared which will subsequently bind to the gene site on the DNA and therefore allow it to be recognised. DNA from the chorionic villi is cut into small fragments by specific enzymes and is then denatured to produce a single strand. The gene probe is then added and it binds with the specific gene, which can then be recognised by means of the radioactivity. This can be used to identify conditions such as α-thalassaemia in which a gene is missing, or for conditions such as sickle cell anaemia where the abnormal sickle cell gene prevents the specific enzymes from cutting up the DNA.

Unfortunately, direct gene probes are only available for a few conditions that are caused by a single gene mutation. Some conditions, for example β-thalassaemia, may be caused by multiple mutations. In such cases, family studies, involving an affected child and its parents, are necessary to determine whether the gene is informative. DNA from each member of the family is broken down into short lengths by specific enzymes, and a specific segment (known as a restriction fragment length polymorphism, RFLP) that is attached to the gene in question is sought. If an RFLP is found in the affected child and one or both of its parents, then this can be sought by DNA analysis of chorionic villi in the next pregnancy.

In some cases where the gene has not been cloned, RFLPs may also be used by searching for a segment of DNA that is closely related to the site where the gene is suspected to be. In these cases, however, there is a risk of misdiagnosis in 2–5% of cases.

Finally, DNA has been used to look for rubella and toxoplasmosis in trophoblastic tissue. Both these conditions may cause severe congenital abnormalities if they cross the placenta, and the finding of viral DNA in chorionic villi appears to be a reliable method of determining whether the virus has infected the fetus.

Enzyme analysis

Most inborn errors of metabolism are autosomal recessive, carrying a one in four chance of affecting the next pregnancy. Increasingly, they are being detected by direct assay of culture of chorionic villi although great care must be taken to avoid maternal contamination. At present, however, they are still largely experimental; results that suggest an unaffected fetus should be backed up by amniocentesis.

CHAPTER TEN
The placenta

LOCATING THE PLACENTA IN EARLY PREGNANCY

With the exception of women undergoing chorion villus sampling (Ch. 9), accurate assessment of placental position is usually attempted for the first time at the routine 16–20 week scan.

Method

The uterus is scanned in its longitudinal axis. The placenta is easily

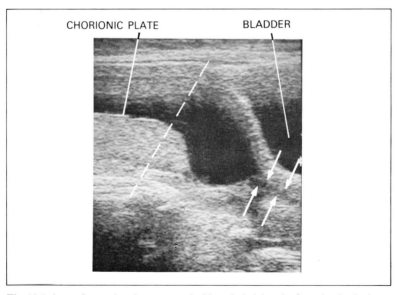

Fig. 10.1 A type I posterior placenta praevia. Note the bright echo from the chorionic plate. The area covered by the bladder is the lower segment, and by projecting this backwards (dotted line) the lower segment can be defined posteriorly. The arrows indicate the cervical canal.

recognised by a stronger echo pattern compared to that of the underlying myometrium. Careful inspection will demonstrate the chorionic plate as a bright linear echo (Fig. 10.1) between the homogeneous echoes of the body of the placenta and the amniotic fluid.

Placenta praevia is a term relating placental position to the lower segment. Before 28 weeks the uterus does not have a true lower segment. If the placenta encroaches on the internal os before 28 weeks it is better to define it as low lying and retain the term 'placenta praevia' until after 28 weeks gestation. In order to determine if the placenta is low lying in early pregnancy the woman should be scanned with a full bladder. Both the internal os and the lower edge of the placenta should be visualised on the same scan. In practice, we do not ask women to attend with a full bladder at the time of the 16–20 week scan as the majority will have an obviously fundal placenta. In a few cases, where a low lying placenta is suspected at the time of the scan, it will be necessary to ask the woman to fill her bladder.

If transvaginal scanning facilities are available this removes the need for a full bladder. In addition, the exact relationship of the lower edge of the placenta to the internal os is more readily appreciated.

Diagnostic pitfalls

The Braxton Hicks contraction

Figure 10.2 demonstrates how the Braxton Hicks contraction may be a trap for the unwary. These contractions cause a 'bunching' up of the myometrium, particularly on the low posterior wall of the uterus, and are easily mistaken for a low posterior placenta (or a fibroid). Examination of the entire uterus will prevent this mistake as the placenta can be recognised elsewhere. Secondly, the lower edge of the placenta should always be sought by keeping the strong linear echo from the chorionic plate in view. Braxton Hicks contractions do not produce this echo. Finally, if there is still real doubt, the woman should be rescanned after a 20 minute period during which time the Braxton Hicks contraction will have disappeared.

Overdistension of the bladder

If the bladder is overfull it compresses the uterus causing the low anterior and low posterior walls to meet, simulating a low lying placenta. This can be excluded by asking the woman to empty her bladder and then rescanning her.

Is localising the placenta at 16–20 weeks gestation worthwhile?

Yes. Approximately 95% of women will have an obviously fundal placenta at this gestation and, therefore, will not have placenta praevia

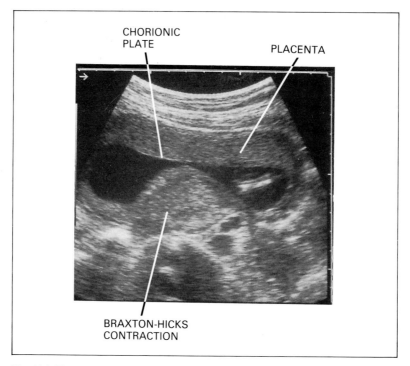

Fig. 10.2 Transverse section of a uterus with an anterior placenta and posterior mass due to a Braxton Hicks contraction. Note the absence of the chorionic plate over the contraction.

in later pregnancy. The remaining 5% will have a low placenta at 16–20 weeks and should therefore be rescanned in the third trimester. One in five of these will have a true placenta praevia.

Obstetric management of the patient with a low lying placenta at 16–20 weeks

If the woman has had no bleeding it is probably only necessary to request a rescan in the third trimester. If the woman has bled or if she has lost several previous pregnancies she may be admitted to hospital or advised to refrain from sexual intercourse.

PLACENTA PRAEVIA

Classification

Figure 10.3 illustrates the two most commonly used classifications of placenta praevia.

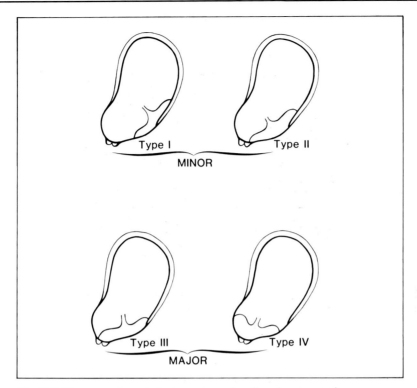

Fig. 10.3 Diagram to illustrate the two systems of grading placenta praevia.

The clinical problem

It is obvious that if the placenta overlies the internal os, vaginal delivery can only occur through the placenta. With the major degrees of placenta praevia life-threatening bleeding will occur when the uterus contracts and the placenta separates. In some cases this will not occur until the woman goes into labour; alternatively it may occur any time during the pregnancy in response to a Braxton Hicks contraction. Women known to have major degrees of placenta praevia are usually kept in hospital (with cross-matched blood permanently available) and are delivered by elective Caesarean section at about 38 weeks (before labour starts) or earlier if they have had a large haemorrhage.

Method of diagnosis

The lower uterine segment unfortunately has no special ultrasonic landmarks but it is obviously important to attempt to define it when placenta praevia is suspected. The woman must have a full bladder which will cover the lower segment anteriorly. The posterior aspect of the lower segment can then be determined by projecting the upper edge of the bladder onto the posterior wall of the uterus (Fig. 10.1). Unless the placenta is quite clearly in the fundus, the internal os and the lower edge of the placenta should be demonstrated on the same scan.

Problems

The most common problem is locating the lower edge of a posterior placenta. The presenting part of the fetus attenuates the ultrasound such that few echoes are obtained from the posterior myometrium. Scanning in from the sides of the uterus may overcome this problem and allow the lower edge of the placenta to be seen. Alternatively, placing the woman in a head down position may displace the presenting part so that the posterior myometrium above the internal os can be visualised. Very rarely, it may be necessary to lift the fetal shoulder to displace the fetal head away from the lower segment. However, if the presenting part is so low in the pelvis that this manoeuvre is necessary, then, even if the placenta reaches to the lower segment, the placenta will not cause a problem with delivery.

Use of a transvaginal probe inserted a few centimetres into the vagina will easily overcome this problem. The higher resolution gained by use of a 6–7.5 MHz transducer together with the fact that the fetal presenting part is no longer in the line of the beam allows clear visualisation of the posterior lower segment. We only recommend transvaginal scanning in women with a questionable low placenta on abdominal scanning as, in our experience, these women are wary of vaginal examinations.

Clinical management of the woman with placenta praevia

If the woman has bled during pregnancy or has a major degree of placenta praevia the obstetrician will advise hospital admission. Two units of blood, correctly cross-matched, will be kept available. Serial scans to monitor fetal growth and placental position will be requested, although fetal growth is rarely affected in women with placenta praevia. The woman with a major degree of placenta praevia will be delivered by Caesarean section at 38 weeks, or before if she has had a sizeable haemorrhage.

Management of women with minor degrees of placenta praevia is not universally agreed upon. The problems are as follows:

1. What to do with women with asymptomatic placenta praevia?

Whilst most obstetricians would advise admission for women with major degrees of placenta praevia, it is probably unnecessary to admit those with minor degrees of placenta praevia if they do not bleed. Bleeding in these women is very unlikely to be life threatening.

2. How reliable is the interpretation of the ultrasound examination?

In skilled hands, ultrasound placentography has a negligible false positive rate. Unfortunately, it is still common practice to anaesthetise the woman at 38 weeks gestation and then to perform a vaginal examination to see if the lower edge of the placenta can be felt and/or made to bleed. If this is the case the woman is delivered by Caesarean section. If not, she is woken up and put into labour.

This is obviously a dangerous practice as occasionally a massive haemorrhage will result. Furthermore, it is not very pleasant for the woman to have to labour whilst suffering the after effects of a general anaesthetic.

Many obstetricians who perform ultrasound have abandoned the grading of placenta praevia and simply report the distance in centimetres of the lower edge of the placenta from the internal os (Fig. 10.4). If the placenta does not reach the internal os the woman is scanned finally at 37–38 weeks gestation in a slightly head down position. If the BPD is below the lower edge of the placenta then she is allowed to await the spontaneous onset of labour. If not she is offered an elective Caesarean section.

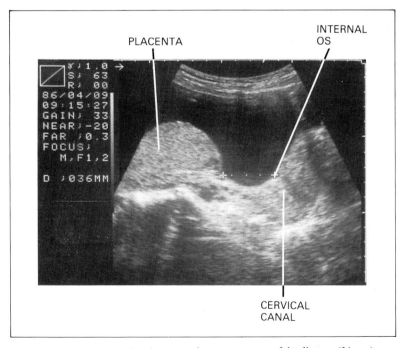

Fig. 10.4 Longitudinal section demonstrating measurement of the distance (36 mm) from the lower edge of the placenta to the internal os.

NORMAL VARIATIONS IN PLACENTAL MORPHOLOGY

1. *Succenturate lobe* (Fig. 10.5)

This is defined as one (or more) accessory lobes of the placenta that is attached to the bulk of the placenta by blood vessels. Making the diagnosis is important as it is possible to have a fundal placenta and a succenturate lobe that is centrally placed over the internal os. These women have the same problems as those with placenta praevia. Very rarely, the intervening vessels may be fetal in origin (vasa praevia) and may rupture during labour. This leads to massive fetal bleeding. Finally, the succenturate lobe may be retained after delivery and may be the source of postpartum haemorrhage or infection.

2. *Placental lakes* (Fig. 10.6)

These lie within the bulk of the placenta and are filled with moving blood. They probably represent the intervillous space in an area lacking fetal villi. They are of no apparent significance.

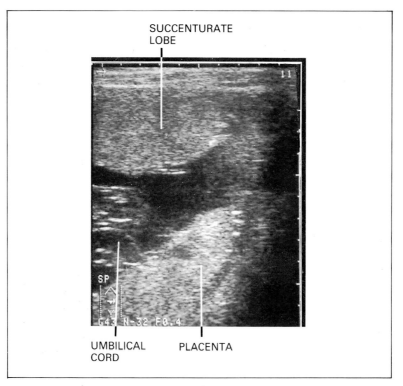

Fig. 10.5 Longitudinal section of a uterus with a posteriorly placed placenta and an anterior succenturate lobe.

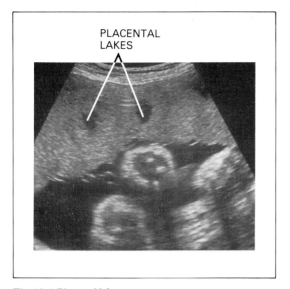

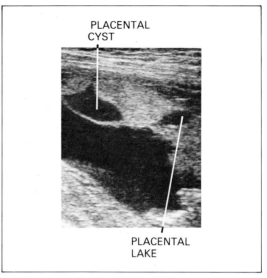

Fig. 10.6 Placental lakes.

Fig. 10.7 A placenta demonstrating both a subchorionic cyst and a placental lake.

3. *Placental cysts* (Fig. 10.7)

These are found immediately beneath the chorionic plate. The smaller ones are blood vessels viewed in cross-section. The larger ones may be distinct entities caused by the deposition of fibrin in the intervillous space. They have no apparent significance.

4. *Highly echogenic areas*

Echogenic areas seen in the placenta in late pregnancy represent normal changes that occur with increasing gestation (see 'Placental grading' below).

PLACENTAL GRADING

This is a classification of the normal changes that occur in the placenta during the course of a pregnancy; it is often known as Grannum grading after its author. Originally it was suggested that a grade III placenta was always associated with mature fetal lungs. This concept has been largely rejected in the United Kingdom and placental grading is rarely used. It is included for completeness and because it illustrates the varying appearances of the normal placenta.

Figure 10.8 illustrates the grading and Figures 10.9–10.11 the ultrasonic changes.

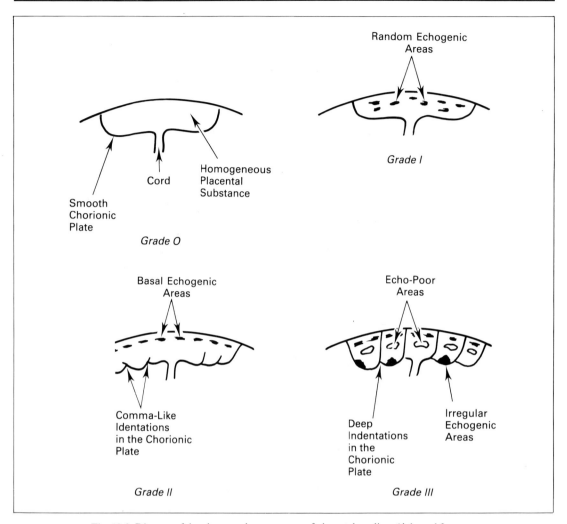

Fig. 10.8 Diagram of the ultrasound appearances of placental grading. (Adapted from Grannum PAT, Berkowitz RL & Hobbins JC (1982) American Journal of Obstetrics and Gynecology 133:915.)

PLACENTAL ABRUPTION

About 3% of the pregnant population will bleed after 28 weeks gestation. Approximately one third of these women will have suffered a placental abruption, in which all or some of the placenta separates from the underlying myometrium before the fetus has been delivered. If this is a major abruption, it is usually clinically apparent because of abdominal pain and a peculiar 'woody hardness' to the uterus. Ultrasound has no place in the diagnosis of major abruption although it may be needed to determine whether the fetus is still alive.

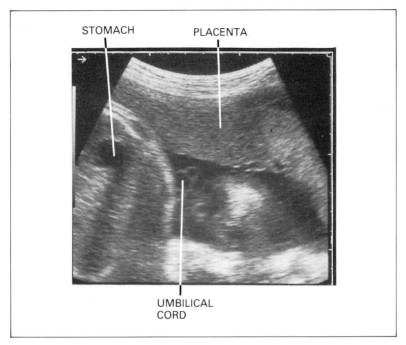

Fig. 10.9 A Grannum grade 0 anterior placenta.

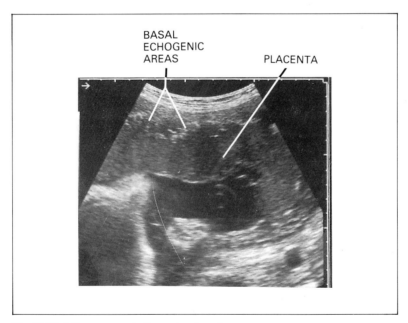

Fig. 10.10 A Grannum grade II anterior placenta.

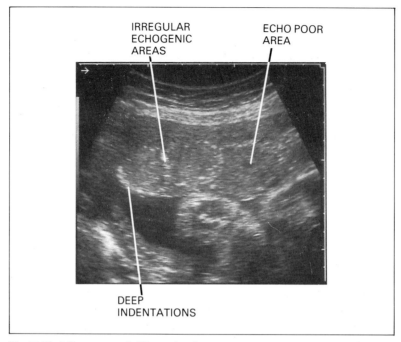

Fig. 10.11 A Grannum grade III anterior placenta.

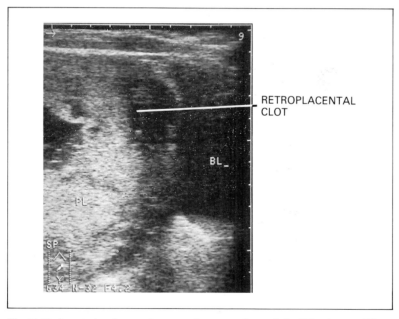

Fig. 10.12 An anterior placenta demonstrating a retroplacental clot (PL: placenta; BL: bladder).

Minor abruptions

These may produce little or no symptoms. The woman presents with slight abdominal pain and/or an antepartum haemorrhage. The diagnosis is difficult to make either clinically or by ultrasound. The main role of ultrasound in these cases is in excluding placenta praevia although occasionally a retroplacental clot may be seen as a hypoechoic area between the placenta and the myometrium (Fig. 10.12). It must be stressed, however, that ultrasound is very unreliable in refuting or confirming the diagnosis of minor abruption.

PLACENTA CIRCUMVALLATA

This literally means a placenta with a ditch around it. Instead of the fetal membranes inserting normally into the edge of the placenta they are inserted a little way along the fetal surface, leaving an area of placenta free of membranes (Fig. 10.13). The site of insertion is usually marked by a depression in the surface of the placenta (hence circumvallata). The membrane-free area tends to separate and bleed but rarely causes more than a little spotting. However, the condition has a high incidence of SGA. It is probably responsible for less than 0.5% of all antepartum haemorrhage but because it cannot be excluded

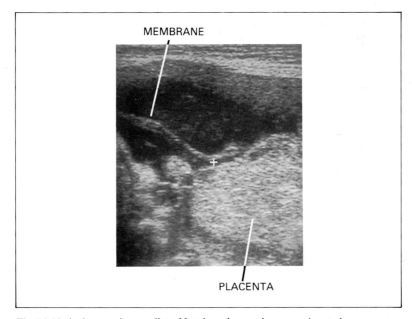

Fig. 10.13 A placenta circumvallata. Note how the membranes are inserted some distance from the placental edge. The cursor (+) indicates the site of insertion.

in cases of undiagnosed APH all women with undiagnosed APH should be serially scanned to exclude SGA.

BLEEDING FROM THE MARGINAL SINUS

This is often a brisk, moderately heavy bleed that is often mistaken clinically for placenta praevia. It is not commonly diagnosed on ultrasound but very occasionally the subsequent clot may be seen (Fig. 10.14).

CHORIOANGIOMA

This is a very rare vascular tumour of the placenta. They vary both in appearance and in size and occasionally appear to be separate from the placenta (Fig. 10.15). They are benign and, if less than 5 cm in diameter, rarely cause a problem. Larger tumours are associated with polyhydramnios and hydrops fetalis.

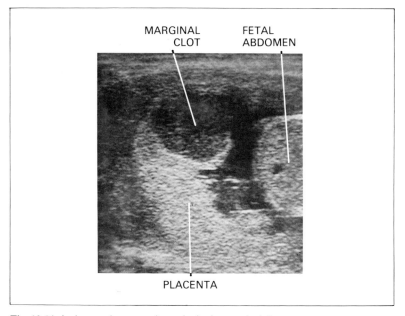

Fig. 10.14 A placenta demonstrating a clot in the marginal sinus.

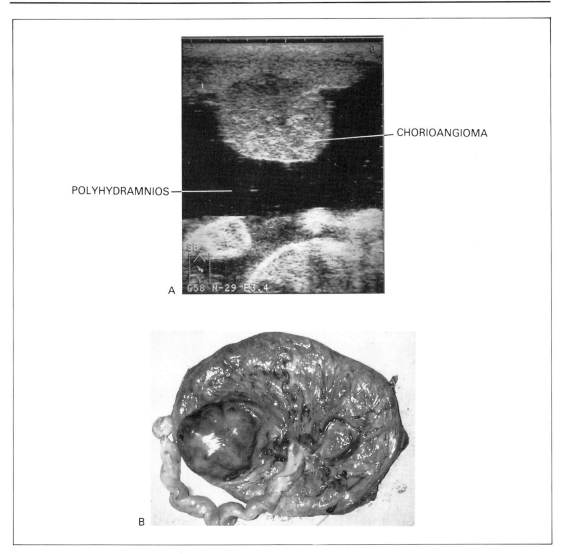

Fig. 10.15 A chorioangioma. (a) Ultrasonic appearance. (b) Histological appearance.

CHAPTER ELEVEN
Normal and abnormal growth

NORMAL GROWTH

The rate of growth of the fetus (and its birthweight) is genetically determined but is modified by environmental factors. For example, the closest associations with birthweight are maternal weight at the start of the pregnancy and mother's own birthweight. This means that even if the father is tall and heavy the size of his child will be modified by the size of the mother. This appears to be nature's attempt to ensure that the fetus is not too large to be delivered by its mother.

Most fetuses show a decline in growth after 38 weeks gestational age. This 'fall off' in growth is related to the overall weight of the 'litter' and the decline can be demonstrated once litter weight achieves 3.2 kg. Thus it occurs at 38 weeks in a singleton, 30 weeks in twins, 27 weeks in triplets and 26 weeks in quadruplets.

ABNORMAL GROWTH

A major aim of antenatal care is to detect the fetus whose growth deviates from a normal pattern. The reasons are as follows:

The large fetus

Fetuses that have excessive growth rates cause difficulties with delivery. The head of a large baby may not be able to pass through its mother's pelvis (cephalopelvic disproportion) or if the head is delivered the shoulders may get stuck (shoulder dystocia). Disproportion causes long, painful labours that commonly end in Caesarean section. The fetus may suffer from lack of oxygen (fetal distress) or may be subject to a difficult instrumental delivery with associated birth trauma. Shoulder dystocia may result in the baby dying during delivery or being delivered with paralysis of the nerves to its face and arms. Breech presentation in large fetuses may mean that the baby is delivered as far as its head, then gets stuck resulting in severe birth asphyxia and trauma or death. Breech babies weighing over 4 kg at birth have three to six times the perinatal mortality rate of breech babies weighing 2.5–4.0 kg; hence the need for an accurate fetal weight estimate in late pregnancy, especially in patients with breech presentations.

Most large infants do not have an apparent cause, but some will be due to maternal diabetes mellitus. Careful serial measurements of growth should be made in this group.

The small fetus

Babies are small because they are born too soon (preterm) or too light in weight (small for dates) or both. Many of the problems of these conditions overlap.

In general, small-for-dates infants can be divided into two groups:

1. Symmetrically small infants

These babies are perfect miniatures, in that they are correctly proportioned but are small (bonsai babies). In most cases they represent the lower end of the normal range, i.e. they are genetically determined to be small and are not, therefore, abnormal. However, some will be small because of chromosomal, infective or environmental factors that exert an influence early in pregnancy (see Table 11.1). Table 11.2 illustrates the problems of symmetrically small babies.

2. Asymmetrically small babies

These infants are long and thin at birth. They have a head size that is appropriate for gestational age but have wasted bodies. They look as

Table 11.1 Causes of intrauterine growth retardation

Symmetrical
Idiopathic
Chromosomal anomalies
TORCH infections
Maternal smoking
Ionising radiation
Heroin addiction
Fetal alcohol syndrome
Chronic maternal undernutrition
Sickle cell disease

Asymmetrical
Idiopathic (probably mostly inadequate placental perfusion)
Proteinuric hypertension
Severe maternal cardiac or renal disease
Multiple gestation

Table 11.2 Problems associated with symmetrical SGA

Chromosomal anomaly
Intrauterine viral infection
Reduced intellect and learning difficulties
Short stature
Increased incidence of death in the first year

though they have been starved. This is true because in most cases their size is the result of 'placental insufficiency'. The placenta effectively supplies the fetus with nourishment and oxygen, and removes waste products. When the placenta begins to fail, its ability to supply nourishment declines before its ability to supply oxygen. Detecting failure of growth is therefore an early warning that the oxygen supply to the fetus will decline in the near future.

All fetuses build up reserves of energy so that they can withstand labour. These reserves are stored as a complex sugar (glycogen) in the fetal liver. During uterine contractions the oxygen supply to the fetus is effectively shut off and the fetus survives these times by using its liver glycogen to supply energy. This decreases its general need for oxygen such that most of the available oxygen can be used by its brain. If the fetus has no glycogen stores then the brain becomes starved of oxygen and 'brain damage' in the form of cerebral palsy or major mental handicap will occur. If the reduction in oxygen to the brain is severe then the fetus will die.

Fetuses that have little or no glycogen stores are those that are preterm and those that are asymmetrically small. In the case of preterm infants, labour occurs before the fetus has been able to complete its stores of glycogen. In asymmetrically small infants the fetus has used its stores of glycogen to allow its brain to continue to grow.

Table 11.3 lists the potential problems of asymmetrically small infants. If they can be delivered before they become short of oxygen then they exhibit 'catch up' growth and are as well grown and intellectually able as appropriately grown babies.

Table 11.3 Problems associated with asymmetrical SGA

Stillbirth
Antenatal and/or perinatal asphyxia, leading to cerebral palsy and/or major mental handicap.
Hypoglycaemia
Hypothermia
Hypocalcaemia
Polycythaemia
Necrotising enterocolitis
Neonatal pulmonary haemorrhage
Premature delivery

Definitions

Low birthweight infants are those that are born with a birthweight of under 2.5 kg. This will include both preterm and small-for-dates infants. This term is still used in the third world where many patients are unsure of the date of their last menstrual period. In parts of the world where routine ultrasound confirmation of gestational age is practised this term is usually replaced by small for dates (SFD) or small for gestational age (SGA).

Small-for-dates or small-for-gestational-age infants are babies with birthweights under the 10th centile for the gestational age at which they are delivered. Ideally, the chart used to decide that they are small should be derived from the population being studied. In practise, however, standard charts are used.

Appropriate-for-gestational-age (AGA) infants are babies born with birthweights between the 10th and the 90th centile for gestational age. Large-for-gestational-age (LGA) infants are babies with birthweights above the 90th centile.

Intrauterine growth retardation (IUGR) is the term applied to an infant whose growth velocity as a fetus was less than expected. It is commonly used as an interchangeable term with either SFD or SGA but this is incorrect. Not all cases of IUGR are SFD. For instance, if the baby was 'programmed' to be 4.5 kg at delivery and was only 3.7 kg it would not be SFD but would be growth retarded and could be expected to have all the problems associated with IUGR. On the other hand, not all SFD fetuses are cases of IUGR. For example, most cases of symmetrical IUGR have no demonstrable cause and probably represent the lower end of the normal range. These infants should not, therefore, be looked upon as growth retarded.

MONITORING GROWTH

In order to assess fetal growth the age of the fetus must be accurately established before 24 weeks gestation. Any fetal organ or part of the fetal body that can be measured serially can have its growth rate studied but in normal fetuses we are only interested in the growth rates of the head and abdomen.

Methods of obtaining the measurements of HC and AC are described in Chapter 5. Figure 11.1 demonstrates changes in the HC and AC with gestational age (the solid lines). These two charts are recommended by the BMUS Ultrasonic Fetal Measurement Survey as being suitable for most populations.

Ideally, all pregnant women should have fetal growth monitored by measurements of HC and AC every 4 weeks, or more frequently if growth deviates from expected lines. This is obviously not feasible for

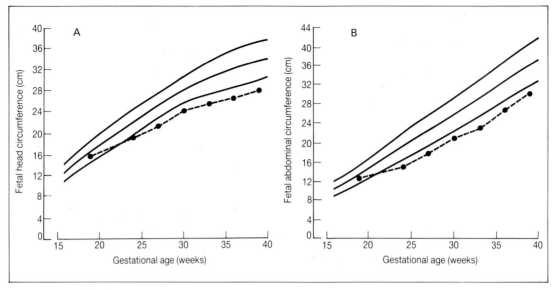

Fig. 11.1 (a) Fetal head circumference and (b) abdominal circumference with increasing gestational age. The solid lines represent the mean and the 95% confidence limits for the original data from which the charts were derived. The dots illustrate the growth pattern of a fetus that demonstrates symmetrical SGA. (HC chart from Hadlock et al (1982) American Journal of Radiology 38: 647–653; AC chart from Deter et al (1982) Journal of Clinical Ultrasound 10: 365–372 reproduced full size in Appendix 5.)

all women. Table 11.4 lists groups of women at particular 'high risk' of having a small or large fetus in which serial measurements of fetal growth are desirable.

At each visit the AC and HC should be measured, the H:A ratio should be calculated, and all three values should be plotted on the appropriate charts. In this fashion, deviations from expected growth patterns can easily be recognised.

Table 11.4 Women at particularly high risk of SGA

Maternal weight less than 10th centile for height (or under 45 kg as a rough guide).
Previous infant with SGA
Maternal vascular disease
 — essential hypertension
 — pregnancy-induced hypertension
 — diabetes mellitus
 — collagen disorders
Maternal cardiac disease that is severe enough to cause maternal polycythaemia
Heavy smokers
Alcoholics and drug addicts
Women with sickle cell disease
Women with recurrent APH
Women with a raised MSAFP but a structurally normal fetus

H:A ratio

This is simply the result of the HC divided by the AC. Figure 11.2 illustrates several H:A ratio charts. The ratio falls with increasing gestational age and is approximately equal to one at 36 weeks gestation. The ratio is mainly of use for differentiating between symmetrical and asymmetrical SGA.

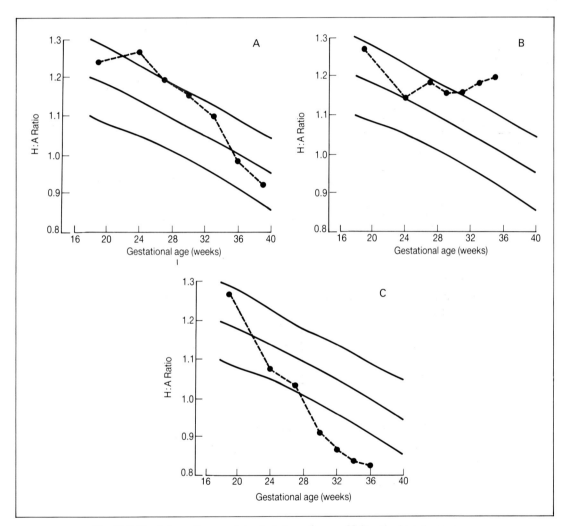

Fig. 11.2 Head circumference: abdominal circumference (H:A) ratio charts (mean ± 2SDs) in cases of altered growth. (a) Symmetrical SGA — most of the observations are within normal limits. (b) Asymmetrical SGA — demonstrating a gradual rise as the growth of the AC becomes static. (c) Macrosomic growth in the fetus of a diabetic mother — here the ratio falls as the growth of the AC rapidly outstrips that of the HC. (H:A ratio charts modified from Campbell S & Thoms A (1977) British Journal of Obstetrics and Gynaecology 84: 165–174.) An H:A ratio chart is reproduced in Appendix 5.

Abdominal Area (AA) and Head Area (HA)

These measurements are used to assess fetal growth but are no better than measurements of HC and AC. Unless the machine has facilities for the automatic computation of area they are difficult to calculate but, in theory, are subject to less errors than measurements of HC and AC. However, if your department uses these measurements and has the appropriate charts available, assessment of fetal growth is possible and reliable using these parameters.

Amniotic fluid volume

A rough assessment of amniotic fluid volume may be made by measuring the largest column of amniotic fluid that can be visualised in a vertical plane. This is usually found between the fetal limbs. Normal values are from 2–8 cm. Figures 11.3–11.5 are examples of normal, increased and decreased amniotic fluid volume.

SYMMETRICAL SGA

Figure 11.1 illustrates a typical woman with symmetrical SGA. The initial ultrasound examination accurately dated the pregnancy so that the deviation from normal growth in later pregnancy cannot be attributed to a problem with 'dates'. Growth is at a normal rate in late pregnancy but is below the 5th centile both for AC and HC. The H:A

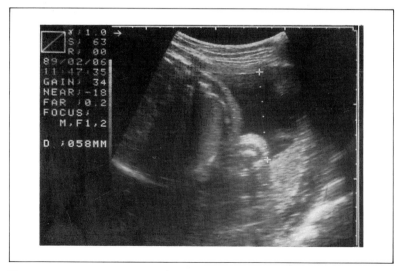

Fig. 11.3 Measurement of an amniotic fluid column. Note the column is measured in the vertical plane and measures 5.8 cm.

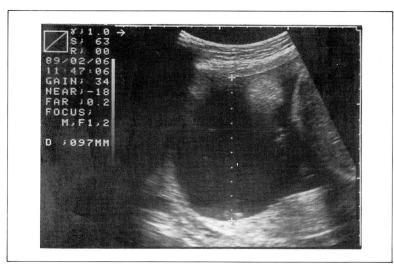

Fig. 11.4 Measurement of an amniotic fluid column (9.7 cm) at 34 weeks gestation in a case of polyhydramnios associated with the macrosomic growth illustrated in Figure 11.7. The woman was a known insulin dependent diabetic.

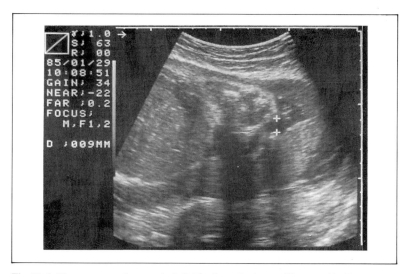

Fig. 11.5 Measurement of an amniotic fluid column in the case illustrated in Figure 11.6. The maximum column visible was only 0.9 cm at 35 weeks.

ratio remains within the normal range, indicating that this is an example of symmetrical SGA.

What to do with cases of symmetrical SGA?

The majority of these babies will be normal but it is very important that the abnormal babies be detected as soon as possible. We suggest the following:

1. A detailed ultrasound examination looking for structural abnormalities including a careful search for minor markers of chromosomal problems (Appendix 3).
2. A subjective assessment of the volume of amniotic fluid. Decreased amniotic fluid and symmetrical SGA may indicate an abnormality of the renal tract.
3. Fortnightly ultrasound measurements of HC and AC made by the same observer on the same machine. At each visit the H:A ratio should be derived because a rise in this ratio may indicate that asymmetrical SGA is being superimposed on symmetrical SGA.
4. Doppler ultrasound measurements (see Ch. 13).

What will the obstetrician do?

If the growth is on or below the 5th centile he will:

a. Search for congenital infections, particularly toxoplasmosis, rubella (German measles), cytomegalovirus and syphilis (this group of infections is often known as TORCH infections).
b. Consider karyotyping the fetus. This can be performed on amniotic fluid obtained via amniocentesis or on fetal blood obtained by cordocentesis. The decision as to whether to karyotype the fetus is difficult but should be encouraged in the presence of minor structural markers (see Appendix 3) or when Doppler studies show an abnormal fetal circulation with normal uteroplacental waveforms (Ch. 13).
c. Look for other causes listed in Table 11.1 and give appropriate advice.
d. Probably await spontaneous labour as these fetuses rarely suffer from fetal distress.

ASYMMETRICAL SGA

Figure 11.6 illustrates the typical findings in a case of asymmetrical SGA. Again, note that the gestational age was established (or confirmed) by an early ultrasound examination. In this case, however, growth of the AC can be seen to slow and eventually stop. Initially, the growth of the HC continues as normal and this is reflected in a rise in the H:A ratio. Eventually, however, the HC also stops growing. As a general guideline, growth of the AC slows 2–3 weeks before that of the HC.

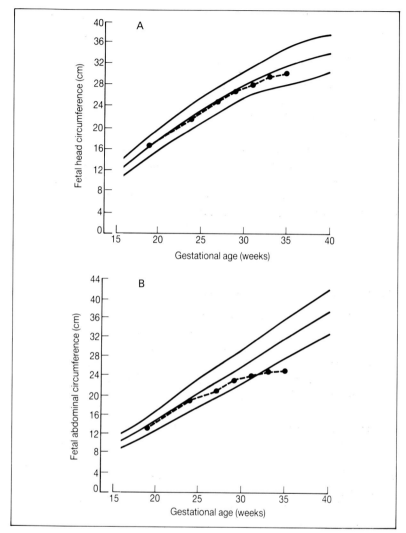

Fig. 11.6 A case of asymmetrical SGA. Note how the growth of the AC tails off whilst the HC continues to grow. Delivery was necessary at 36 weeks because of oligohydramnios and loss of end-diastolic frequencies in the umbilical artery and fetal aorta. (HC chart from Hadlock et al (1982) American Journal of Radiology 38: 647–653; AC chart from Deter et al (1982) Journal of Clinical Ultrasound 10: 365–372 reproduced full size in Appendix 5.)

What to do with cases of asymmetrical SGA?

As these are the women in which timely delivery will prevent perinatal death and handicap, careful monitoring is necessary.

1. Growth should be serially monitored by HC, AC and H:A ratio every two weeks by the same observer on the same machine.

Monitoring growth on a weekly basis is not reliable as the error in measurement is greater than the weekly growth increment (but less than that of the fortnightly increment). Weekly measurements may produce errors in both directions, i.e. they may suggest normal growth in the absence of growth, or reduced growth when growth is normal.

2. Make an estimate of the volume of amniotic fluid. Asymmetrically growth-retarded fetuses with oligohydramnios have a greater incidence of perinatal death or handicap than those with normal volumes of amniotic fluid.

3. Observe the fetus to ensure that it is exhibiting movement and breathing movements (see below).

4. Perform Doppler ultrasound examinations (Ch. 13).

What will the obstetrician do?

a. *If the woman has hypertension or the fetal AC has stopped growing he will admit her to hospital.*

b. *He will start intensive fetal surveillance by monitoring*:
   — Fetal movements. Mother will be asked to keep a record of the number of times her baby kicks her, usually on a Cardiff 'count to ten' chart. Any decrease in activity means further study is needed by means of a cardiotocograph.
   — Cardiotocography (CTG). This is an electronic recording of the fetal heart rate against uterine activity and fetal movements. A poor CTG gives warning that the fetus is becoming short of oxygen and so should be delivered.
   — Fetal activity. This means that the fetus will be observed with real-time ultrasound in order to note the presence or absence of fetal movements (FMs) and fetal breathing movements (FBMs). As general guidelines, a fetus that demonstrates an abundance of FMs and FBMs is not suffering from lack of oxygen.

Table 11.5 The biophysical profile. (From Manning F A, Baskett T F, Morrison I and Lange I (1981) American Journal of Obstetrics and Gynaecology 140: 289, with kind permission of the editor and publishers.)

Parameter	Score 2	Score 0
Heart rate reactivity	Two or more accelerations in 40 minutes	Less than two accelerations
Fetal movement	More than three gross body movements in 30 minutes	Less than three in a 30 minute period
Fetal breathing movements (FBM)	At least 30 seconds sustained FBM in 30 minutes	Less than 30 seconds sustained FBM
Amniotic fluid	More than 1 cm pocket	Less than 1 cm pocket
Fetal tone	Closed fist or a flexion to extension movement	Neither

Unfortunately, absence of FMs or FBMs is more difficult to interpret; healthy fetuses may not breathe for periods of up to 2 hours and may not move for up to 40 minutes. The fetus is at its most active one hour after the mother has eaten; this is obviously the best time to study them. Many schemes have been devised but the biophysical profile illustrated in Table 11.5 is often used. The use of several parameters of 'fetal wellbeing' decreases the risk of a false positive result.
— Doppler ultrasound examinations (see Ch. 13).

c. *He will deliver the baby if:*
  — The CTG and/or the studies on fetal activity suggest the fetus is becoming short of oxygen.
  — The umbilical artery shows absence of end-diastolic frequencies in a fetus of more than 28 weeks gestation.
  — The fetal HC has not grown for three weeks or more. This is an arbitrary limit but it is thought that the fetus has little to gain by remaining in utero after this time and that sudden death is likely.
  — Fetal maturity is reached and the cervix is favourable. In general, the fetus is considered mature at 37 weeks but delivery may be considered from 34 weeks onwards if growth is impaired. The state of the cervix needs to be assessed because if the cervix is 'ripe' (soft and partially open) this indicates that it would be easy to induce labour. If the cervix is unfavourable (hard and closed) induction of labour is likely to fail and delivery will have to be by Caesarean section.
  — The woman's blood pressure becomes uncontrollable.

SCREENING FOR SGA

As not all women can have serial ultrasound examinations, some form of screening must be carried out. Screening in this instance is defined as the recognition of a subgroup of women from the general pregnant population that is at high risk of having an SGA infant. Although the groups of women listed in Table 11.4 are at high risk of having SGA infants, 80% or more SGA infants are born to women without such risk factors.

At each antenatal visit the obstetrician assesses the size of the uterus and the fetus by palpating the abdomen. However, this is highly inaccurate as even the best obstetricians will detect no more than 50% of the small babies. Furthermore, for every three who were thought to be carrying an SGA fetus, only one fetus will actually be SGA. However, any fetus thought to be small clinically should have a careful ultrasound examination.

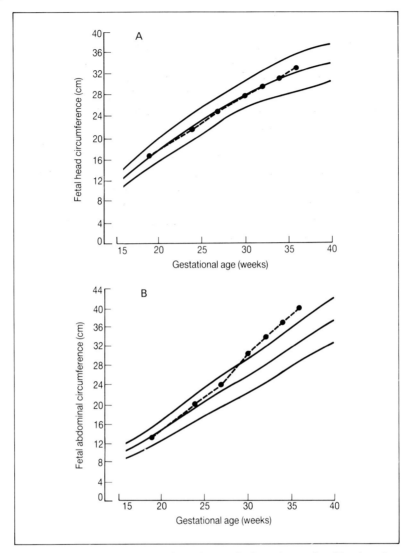

Fig. 11.7 A case of macrosomia in a fetus of an insulin dependent mother. Note how the growth of the AC accelerates from about 28 weeks onwards. (HC chart from Hadlock et al (1982) AJR 38: 647–653; AC chart from Deter et al (1982) Journal of Clinical Ultrasound 10: 365–372.)

Various attempts have been made to screen for SGA with ultrasound and the simplest is by measurement of the fetal AC at 32–36 weeks gestation. This will detect approximately 85% of SGA fetuses. We should suggest that any fetus with an AC of less than 25.0 cm at 32 weeks, 29.0 cm at 34 weeks or 30.5 cm at 36 weeks should have the HC measured and H:A ratio calculated. The fetus should then be measured serially.

GROWTH ACCELERATION

The finding of a large AC (on or above the 90th centile) or of a fetus with accelerated growth (Fig. 11.7) should suggest the possibility of maternal diabetes mellitus. This is particularly so if there is associated polyhydramnios (amniotic column of more than 8 cm) and a large (more than 4 cm thick) placenta. The obstetrician will exclude or confirm the diagnosis by performing a glucose tolerance test.

If the woman is known to have diabetes mellitus a detailed scan to exclude structural anomalies should be performed at 18–20 weeks followed by a scan at 20–22 weeks to exclude a cardiac anomaly. Serial scans of growth should then be performed on a monthly basis. This may be increased to fortnightly if growth deviates from the expected rate. Excessive growth, especially if accompanied by polyhydramnios, suggests poor control of maternal diabetes.

CHAPTER TWELVE
Ultrasound in late pregnancy including fetal weight estimation

We have previously emphasised that gestational age can only be accurately established by ultrasound before 24 weeks postmenstrual age. After this time the errors in predicting fetal age increase markedly with increasing gestation. Moreover, if the measurements are reduced, it is almost impossible to distinguish between symmetrical growth retardation and a 'dates' problem (see 'Late bookers', Ch. 5).

INDICATIONS

Indications for ultrasound examination after 24 weeks are:

- 'High risk' women
- The clinical suspicion of SGA (see Ch. 11)
- A low lying placenta diagnosed at the early scan (see Ch. 10)
- The clinical suspicion of placenta praevia (see Ch. 10)
- Fetal presentation
- Late indicators of potential fetal abnormality
- Fetal weight estimates.

All women having ultrasound examination after 24 weeks should have the BPD, HC and AC measured and the H:A ratio calculated (see Ch. 5) irrespective of the reason for referral. These measurements should be graphically presented. The placental site and fetal presentation should also be noted. Where serial examinations are indicated they should commence from 26 weeks gestation and should be repeated every four weeks providing fetal growth is normal. The management of abnormal growth is covered in Chapter 11.

'HIGH RISK' WOMEN

This is a descriptively poor but commonly used clinical term. It would be more helpful to expand the term to include the condition of which the fetus is at risk. Such conditions include:

SGA fetus (see Table 11.4)

Preterm labour

Most preterm deliveries occur in women who do not have a recognisable risk factor for preterm labour. However, preterm labour is more likely to occur in women who have had a previous preterm infant, those with cervical incompetence, those with polyhydramnios, those with multiple pregnancies and those with maternal diabetes mellitus. It is reasonable to offer serial scans to these women so that if preterm labour occurs a recently performed fetal weight estimation will be available. The decision as to whether to attempt tocolysis (suppression of labour) largely depends upon an accurate knowledge of both the gestational age and the fetal weight. For example, this knowledge is very useful in deciding where delivery should occur. As a general guideline, a fetus that is older than 34 weeks and weighs more than 2.5 kg could safely be managed by a unit that does not have a neonatal intensive care facility. If labour occurs in a woman carrying a younger, lighter fetus she should be transferred to a hospital where such facilities are available.

Preterm labour is more common in pregnancies complicated by fetal abnormalities. These should be carefully sought, especially if the fetus is presenting by the breech. The presence of a nonviable structural abnormality may prevent a Caesarean section.

Placental abruption

Major placental abruptions cannot be predicted by ultrasound. Repeated episodes of abdominal pain and/or vaginal bleeding may suggest recurrent minor abruptions. The resultant retroplacental clots may not be visible on ultrasound but serial examinations are advised as the fetus is at increased risk of being small for gestational age.

Raised MSAFP

Women with raised MSAFP but whose fetus is structurally normal have an approximate six-fold increase in their chances of miscarriage, preterm delivery and of giving birth to a small-for-gestational-age infant. These women should therefore have serial ultrasound. Doppler waveforms from the uteroplacental circulation appear to have a predictive role in these circumstances (see Ch. 13).

Common specific obstetric conditions that carry increased fetal risk

Hypertensive diseases of pregnancy

These women commonly have small-for-gestational-age fetuses. If the hypertension is complicated by proteinuria then they also have an increased risk of placental abruption.

Multiple pregnancy

These women are at increased risk of poor growth in one or both fetuses, polyhydramnios, preterm delivery and placenta praevia. If routine ultrasound is offered at 16–20 weeks all multiple pregnancies should be detected. As the incidence of fetal abnormality is increased in twins — especially monozygotic twins — these women should have an anomaly scan at 18–20 weeks and a detailed cardiac scan at 22–24 weeks.

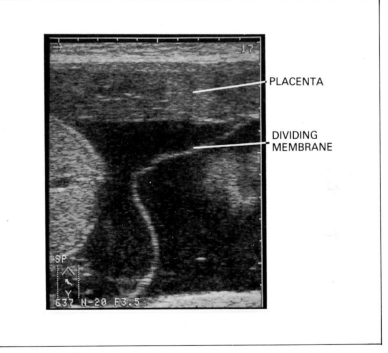

Fig. 12.1 The dividing membrane in dizygotic twins at 24 weeks gestation.

Zygosity in twin pregnancies can be determined by the following means:

1. *Placental sites*. The finding of two separate placental sites indicates dizygotic twins in the vast majority of cases.

2. *Fetal gender*. If the fetuses are of different sex they are dizygotic twins.

3. *The thickness of the dividing membrane*. Dizygotic twins have a four layered membrane (two amnions and two chorions) which is very obvious on ultrasound (Fig. 12.1). Most monozygotic twins have a two layered membrane (two amnions) which appears thin (Fig. 12.2) but in about 6% no membrane is seen as the twins are monoamniotic.

The thickness of the membrane is a reliable guide, especially in the first two trimesters, but errors occur in the form of attributing dizygosity to monozygotic twins.

Twins of the same sex with a single placenta indicate a 70% probability of monozygosity; with two placentae, the probability is reduced to 15%.

All multiple pregnancies should be scanned at least monthly from 24 weeks gestation and the HC and AC (together with the H:A ratio) should be plotted. Figure 12.3 illustrates discordant fetal growth which

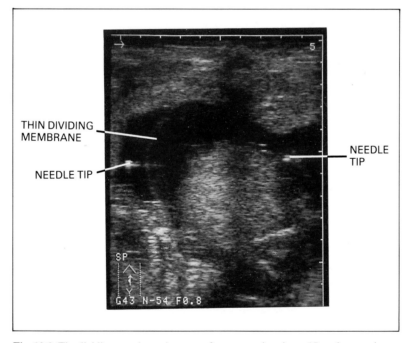

Fig. 12.2 The dividing membrane in a case of monozygotic twins at 17 weeks gestation. Note how it is difficult to visualise compared to that in Figure 12.1. This image was recorded at the time of twin amniocentesis.

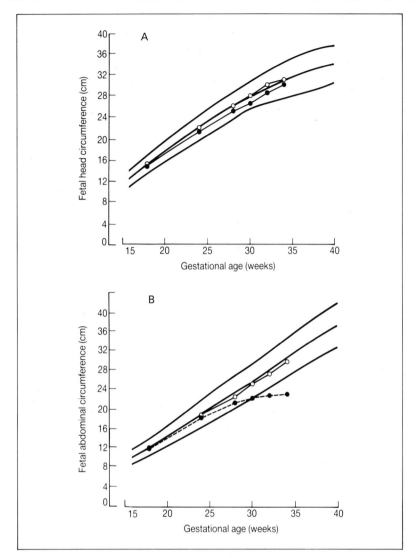

Fig. 12.3 Discordant growth in a twin pregnancy (bold lines represent mean and 95% confidence limits). (a) Normal growth of the fetal head circumferences. (b) Fall off of growth of the fetal abdomen in the second twin.

is only observed in about 10% of all cases of twins but is an indication to repeat the scans fortnightly.

Discordant growth is seen in the following circumstances:

1. *The twin–twin transfusion syndrome*. This is almost entirely a problem of monozygosity. The severity of the situation varies according to the nature of the vascular connections. At its least severe it produces minimal impairment of growth. At its most severe it produces anaemia

and hydrops fetalis in the smaller twin and polycythaemia in the other as blood is shunted from the smaller to the larger twin. In these situations it is not uncommon to encounter acute polyhydramnios and many such pregnancies are lost before 26 weeks gestation.

2. *Disparity in size and growth*. About 10% of twins will be different sizes at 18–20 weeks gestation and gestational age should be ascribed based upon the measurements obtained from the larger twin. The smaller twin usually grows at a normal rate.

Impairment of growth may also be seen after 28 weeks gestation and in such cases it is usually of the asymmetrical type. Management is as for a singleton (Ch. 11). Only rarely will the clinician have to decide between very preterm delivery, in an attempt to save the smaller twin, or allowing the pregnancy to continue to improve the maturity of the well grown twin hence sacrificing the smaller twin.

Higher multiple pregnancies should, in addition, have detailed anomaly scans and serial growth scans. Decisions concerning delivery can be complex because impaired growth is common in one or more fetuses.

Maternal diabetes mellitus

These women carry a risk of fetal abnormalities that is approximately three times that of the normal population; these fetuses should therefore have detailed anomaly scans to exclude structural and cardiac abnormalities. These women are also at increased risk of hypertensive disease of pregnancy (particularly pre-eclampsia), macrosomia, polyhydramnios, preterm delivery and growth retardation, so serial ultrasound is indicated (Ch. 11).

Other maternal medical problems

Women with any serious medical problem should be offered serial ultrasound examinations to assess fetal growth. Apart from hypertensive disease the commonest conditions encountered are maternal cardiac or renal disease.

FETAL PRESENTATION

It should rarely be necessary to request an ultrasound examination for fetal presentation; exceptions include extreme maternal obesity or women with multiple fibroids.

If the presentation is not cephalic the ultrasonographer should exclude placenta praevia, a cervical fibroid or an ovarian tumour as a possible cause. Persistent breech or transverse lies may be associated with such fetal abnormalities as fetal goitre or iniencephaly.

Fetal weight estimates should be reported in women with breech or transverse presentations after 34 weeks gestation (see later).

LATE INDICATORS OF POTENTIAL FETAL ANOMALY

All the indicators for a detailed anomaly scan listed in Table 6.1 will still apply if the woman books late in pregnancy. A detailed anomaly scan should also be performed on women who develop polyhydramnios, those in whom a symmetrically small-for-gestational-age fetus is diagnosed and those with a persistently abnormal lie. Most abnormalities diagnosed in late pregnancy do not occur in these categories but are detected by the observant ultrasonographer during routine examination.

FETAL WEIGHT ESTIMATION

This may be requested in cases of:

- Preterm labour (see above)
- Breech presentation and occasionally in unstable or transverse lie
- Small-for-gestational-age fetus in which early delivery is being considered (see Ch. 11)
- Maternal medical conditions which will be improved by delivery, for example progressive deterioration of renal function because of pregnancy-induced hypertension
- Multiple pregnancy (see above)
- Maternal diabetes mellitus. Infants of diabetic mothers may develop macrosomia which may cause a difficult, prolonged labour and/or difficulties with delivery. Infants weighing over 4.5 kg are particularly prone to shoulder dystocia and consideration should be given to delivery by Caesarean section
- An operable fetal abnormality that is compatible with life but which is deteriorating. For example, hydronephrosis.

Method

The estimation of fetal weight involves errors of up to 160 g per kg of fetal weight and these errors should be appreciated by both the ultrasonographer and the referring clinician. Formulae that involve the measurement of two fetal parameters are about 5% more accurate than those which involve only one parameter, whilst the addition of a third parameter improves the estimation by about a further 1%.

In situations where the BPD and AC can be accurately measured we recommend their use in fetal weight estimation as shown in Appendix 6. In late pregnancy, however, the fetal head may be engaged or, if the presentation is breech, the shape of the head may be dolichocephalic making measurement of the BPD unreliable. In these situations we use measurements of AC and FL (see Appendix 6).

CHAPTER THIRTEEN
Doppler ultrasound

INTRODUCTION

Doppler ultrasound waveforms may be acquired by two means:

- Continuous wave equipment
- Pulsed Doppler equipment. This usually combines real-time imaging with pulsed wave Doppler (duplex, pulsed Doppler) and may also include colour flow mapping.

Chapter 16 explains the differences between the two Doppler systems. Continuous wave Doppler equipment is usually purchased as stand-alone equipment but may be duplexed to existing real-time equipment. It costs approximately £10 000 and is being used increasingly in obstetric practice. Pulsed Doppler equipment costs upwards of £75 000 and its use tends to be confined to research workers or regional referral centres.

CONTINUOUS WAVE DOPPLER EQUIPMENT

Most commonly, continuous wave equipment is used without concurrent real-time imaging facilities and its use in obstetrics is therefore limited to acquiring waveforms from the umbilical artery and the uteroplacental vessels. Although waveforms from other vessels such as the fetal aorta may occasionally be obtained they cannot be produced reliably without pulsed Doppler equipment.

UMBILICAL ARTERY WAVEFORMS

Means of acquiring the signal

Ideally the equipment should be designed specifically for obstetric purposes, as cardiovascular equipment has high power output levels. If your machine has a choice of probes select a 4 MHz probe. Set the vessel wall filter (also known as the thump filter) to 50 Hz, the frequency range to 4 KHz and the sweep speed to 5 m/s. Ensure the balance knob is exactly at its mid-position and that the gain control is set at about 50% of maximum. Turn the volume control on the loudspeaker up so that on gentle tapping the probe produces a loud noise. If your machine has an automatic maximum frequency follower it should be set to average three waveforms and ideally should be turned off until you are happy that the waveforms on the screen are ideal.

Place the probe in the middle of the woman's abdomen, just below the umbilicus. Slowly search the uterus with the probe until the signal seen in Figure 13.1 is displayed on the screen. Most operators learn to hear the signal long before the visual display is seen. Making fine movements of the probe use your eyes and ears to acquire a signal that has a good signal-to-noise ratio. This means that the waveform has a clear outline and that there is not a second waveform from another vessel superimposed. Alter the gain settings to help reduce noise and ensure that the waveform fills about two-thirds of the screen by altering the frequency range setting. Ideally, try to record the umbilical vein in the opposite channel as a continuous smooth signal (Fig. 13.1) as this demonstrates the absence of fetal breathing or movement, both of which can alter the height of the Doppler shifted frequencies (Fig. 13.2).

If the machine has a maximum frequency follower, turn this back on and freeze the image when the automatic calculations appear on the screen. Examine the three waveforms that the machine has chosen to ensure that they are free from substantial noise and that the machine

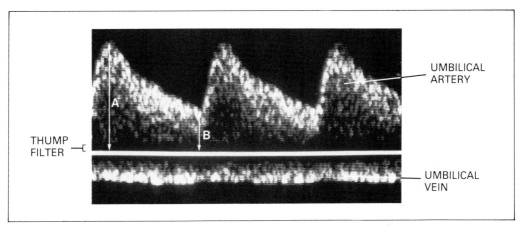

Fig. 13.1 A continuous wave recording of a normal umbilical artery and vein at 32 weeks gestation. The vein appears in the opposite channel to the artery as flow within it is away from the transducer. (A = maximum systolic frequency, B = minimum end-diastolic frequency)

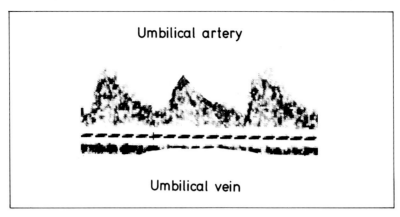

Fig. 13.2 A continuous wave recording of an umbilical artery and vein demonstrating the effects of fetal breathing. The vein does not show a steady continuous pattern.

has correctly chosen the maximum systolic point and the least frequency in end-diastole (Fig. 13.1).

If the machine does not have a maximum frequency follower then freeze the waveforms on the screen and use the cursors to measure the maximum systolic frequency and the minimum frequency recorded in end-diastole (Fig. 13.1).

Methods of measuring and reporting the waveform

The waveform obtained is usually characterised by an index that describes the maximum frequency outline (Fig. 13.3). These indices allow comparisons between waveforms. The umbilical artery is most commonly reported in terms of the A:B ratio (also known as the systolic:diastolic or S:D ratio). Use the light pen or rollerball apparatus

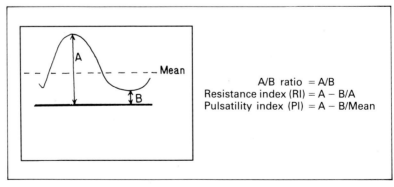

Fig. 13.3 A schematic waveform showing how the common indices that are applied to the maximum frequency outline are obtained.

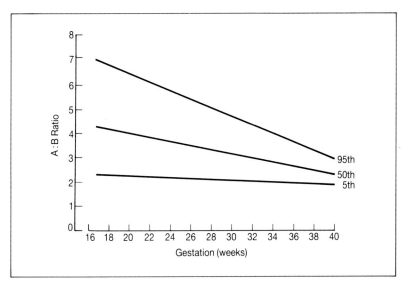

Fig. 13.4 The data reference range for the A:B ratio from the umbilical artery. (This chart is produced full size in Appendix 5.)

to measure the height of the systolic peak in KHz and then measure the height of the minimum frequency in end-diastole, also in KHz. The A:B ratio is derived from the average of at least three and preferably five waveforms. We suggest that you plot this on a data reference range (Fig. 13.4) and then, as well as reporting the A:B ratio, you should comment if this value lies outside the data reference range. Situations where no frequencies are recorded in end-diastole (Fig. 13.5) are best reported in words, viz: 'End-diastolic frequencies were absent in the umbilical artery.' Rarely, frequency in end-diastole may appear in the opposite channel (Fig. 13.6) and this should also be reported in words: 'The umbilical artery demonstrated reversal of frequencies in end-diastole.'

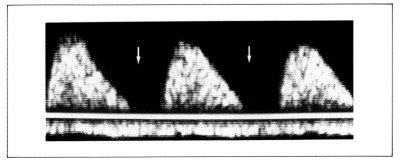

Fig. 13.5 A continuous wave recording of an umbilical artery and vein demonstrating loss of diastolic frequencies in the umbilical artery (arrows).

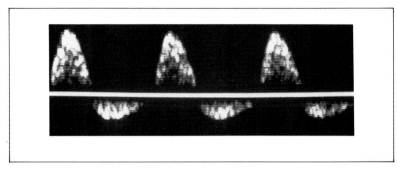

Fig. 13.6 A continuous wave recording of an umbilical artery demonstrating reversed flow. The frequencies seen in the reverse channel are from the umbilical artery and in this situation a venous signal should not be sought as it may obscure the reversed frequencies.

The justification for the use of words rather than ratios is given in Chapter 16 but essentially all three ratios illustrated in Figure 13.3 are of no use when end-diastolic frequencies are lost and only the pulsatility index (see p. 283) can cope with reversed frequencies. As these situations carry major significance (see clinical interpretation) you should institute an internal quality check to avoid artifactual loss of end-diastolic frequencies. We suggest that in order to say that end-diastolic frequencies are truly absent you must obtain a signal from two separate sites on the uterus on two successive days.

Problems in acquiring and interpreting the waveforms

Artifactual loss of end-diastolic frequencies

This may be due to:

1. A high angle between the ultrasound beam and the vessel that results in very low frequencies disappearing below the height of the vessel wall filter. If end-diastolic frequencies appear absent you should reduce the vessel wall filter to its lowest setting (usually 50 Hz), or remove it if possible. Then you should alter the angle of the probe relative to the maternal abdomen and if end-diastolic frequencies are still absent you should then attempt to obtain the signal from a different site within the uterus as this is likely to result in a different angle of insonation. You should also ensure that the fetus is not breathing by demonstrating a smooth waveform from the umbilical vein in the opposite channel. We do not report absence of end-diastolic frequencies until this has been demonstrated on two successive days. The alternative is to submit the woman to a duplex, pulsed Doppler examination (see below).

2. Fetal breathing movements. These cause wild fluctuations in the signal from the umbilical artery and are readily recognisable by being

unable to demonstrate a steady state in the umbilical vein that is recorded in the other channel (Fig. 13.2). After a little practice, they can also be recognised from the arterial signal. The only course to take if the fetus is breathing is to wait until this stops.

Failure to obtain a signal

This may be due to:

1. Incorrect machine settings. This is usually recognised by hearing a signal that is not displayed on the screen. First check that the frequency range is not too high or low — 4 MHz is a good starting point. If the screen is still blank then turn up the gain slowly. If the screen is saturated with white noise then turn the gain down slowly until the waveform appears. If there is still no visual signal then ensure that the balance setting is not turned to one extreme such that one channel of the spectrum analyser is obliterated.
2. Fetal death.
3. Maternal obesity.
4. Oligohydramnios.

In the latter three situations, use a real-time transducer to check that the fetus is still alive and then to locate a loop of cord. Mark the spot on the maternal abdomen with a finger and then replace the real-time transducer with the Doppler probe. You cannot undertake real-time imaging and acquire Doppler signals simultaneously, as the signals interfere with each other. In pulsed Doppler machines the real-time image is usually frozen when the Doppler signal is being acquired (see Ch. 16).

Indications for umbilical artery waveforms

Currently only the following indications have been shown to have any validity:

- Assessment and continued monitoring of the fetus that has been demonstrated to be small for gestational age on real-time ultrasound
- Assessment of the fetus of a mother with systemic lupus erythematosus (SLE)
- Assessment of differing sizes or growth patterns in twins
- In conjunction with uteroplacental waveforms in the assessment of oligohydramnios.

Contra-indications to umbilical artery waveforms

Umbilical artery waveforms are of little or no value as a screening test for the small-for-gestational-age fetus and do not appear to predict unexplained antepartum stillbirths. They are also not predictive of placental abruption.

The role of umbilical artery waveforms is not established in fetuses of insulin dependent diabetics and fetal death has been reported within 24 hours of obtaining normal umbilical artery waveforms from the fetuses of such women. The place of umbilical artery waveforms in antepartum haemorrhage and preterm labour or rupture of the membranes is unknown.

Interpretation of the waveforms

1. In the absence of an acute incident such as a placental abruption, a small-for-gestational-age fetus with normal umbilical artery waveforms will not develop loss of end-diastolic frequencies within a 7 day period, so that monitoring may be performed weekly.

2. Only 10% of fetuses that are demonstrated to be asymmetrically small for gestational age on real-time ultrasound will demonstrate loss of end-diastolic frequencies at any time during their pregnancy.

3. Loss of end-diastolic frequencies is associated with an 85% chance that the fetus will be hypoxic in utero and a 50% chance that it will also be acidotic.

4. The finding of a symmetrically small fetus with absent end-diastolic frequencies in the umbilical artery but with normal uteroplacental waveforms suggests the possibility of a primary fetal cause for the growth retardation such as a chromosomal abnormality or a TORCH virus infection.

5. Fetuses demonstrating absence of end-diastolic frequencies but which are managed along standard clinical lines have a 40% chance of dying and at least a 25% morbidity rate from necrotising enterocolitis, haemorrhage or coagulation failure after birth. The time between loss of end-diastolic frequencies and fetal death appears to differ for each fetus. Following loss of end-diastolic frequencies there are no other reliable changes in the waveform that help in deciding when to deliver the baby.

6. Reversed frequencies in end-diastole are only observed in a few fetuses prior to death. This finding should be considered as a pre-terminal condition; few if any, fetuses will survive without some form of therapeutic intervention.

7. Loss of end-diastolic frequencies precedes changes in the cardiotocograph by some 7–42 days in fetuses that have been shown to be small for gestational age on real-time ultrasound. In the absence of maternal hypertension many centres would now monitor small-for-gestational-age fetuses solely with Doppler ultrasound. The occurrence of CTG decelerations not related to contractions, together with absent end-diastolic frequencies, carries an extremely poor prognosis.

Current recommendations

It is probably reasonable for the clinician to deliver all small-for-gestational-age fetuses that present with absent (or reversed) end-diastolic frequencies after 28 weeks gestation. In units with neonatal intensive care facilities the perinatal mortality for infants that are more than 28 weeks gestations is less than 10% with about a 6% chance of handicap in the survivors. If these fetuses are managed along standard clinical lines a mortality rate of about 40% with a 25% chance of severe handicap can be expected.

At less than 28 weeks gestation these fetuses should probably be referred to a regional centre for detailed studies of the fetal circulation and possibly cordocentesis, with an aim to therapy that may improve fetal oxygenation and growth.

UTEROPLACENTAL WAVEFORMS

Means of acquiring the signal

Initially, uteroplacental waveforms were acquired from the uterine or arcuate artery by means of duplex, pulsed Doppler ultrasound. This allowed real-time images to be interlaced with the Doppler waveforms; therefore, even if the uteroplacental vessel could not be imaged, it was possible to say with confidence that the signal originated from a vessel within the uterus. As it is not always possible to determine whether these waveforms arise from the uterine artery or the arcuate artery they

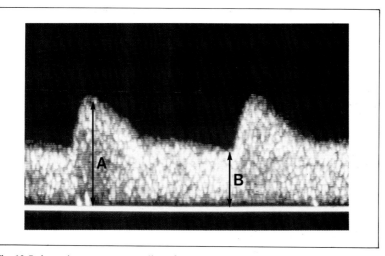

Fig. 13.7 A continuous wave recording of a uteroplacental waveform from a normal pregnancy after 24 weeks gestation. (A = maximum systolic frequency, B = minimum end-diastolic frequency.) RI = 0.38.

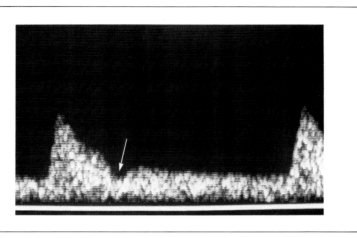

Fig. 13.8 A continuous wave recording of a uteroplacental waveform from a pregnancy complicated by proteinuric hypertension. RI = 0.72. The arrow indicates the dicrotic notch which is not seen in the normal waveform. This notch and the high RI indicate an increased peripheral resistance and reduced blood flow into the intervillous space.

are commonly referred to as uteroplacental waveforms. With experience it was realised that such waveforms have a characteristic pattern in both normal and abnormal pregnancies (Figs 13.7 & 13.8).

Method

Set up your machine as described under 'Umbilical artery waveforms'. Imagine the shape of the uterus within the maternal abdomen and then search the lower, outer quadrant on each side until you hear, then see, the characteristic waveform (Fig. 13.7). Alternatively, locate the anterior superior iliac spine and then move the probe a few centimetres medially. Angle the probe towards the pubic symphysis. When the waveform is seen, alter the frequency range on the equipment until the waveform fills about two-thirds of the height of the screen. If the machine has a maximum frequency follower, turn it back on and freeze the image when the automatic calculations are displayed. Examine the three waveforms that the machine has chosen to ensure that they are free from substantial noise and that the machine has correctly chosen the maximum systolic point and the least frequency in end-diastole. If the machine does not have a maximum frequency follower then freeze the image and measure the maximum systolic frequency and minimum frequency in end-diastole as illustrated in Figure 13.7.

How to report uteroplacental waveforms

Loss of end-diastolic frequencies is extremely rare in the uteroplacental circulation so a simple index such as the A:B ratio or resistance index (see p. 224) is sufficient. There is no consensus as to which ratio should be used. In addition to the A:B ratio and the resistance index, the pulsatility index and the B:A ratio have been used. We suggest that you use the resistance index as it reminds you (and your clinical colleagues) that the waveforms are a reflection of the peripheral resistance to the blood flow into the intervillus space.

As with umbilical arteries we recommend that you store at least 10 waveforms in the machine's memory and measure the three with the highest signal to noise ratio.

Record the waveforms from both sides of the uterus. We suggest that you report them as follows:

a. *Low resistance pattern* — both sides have an RI < 0.58
b. *High resistance pattern* — both sides have an RI > 0.58

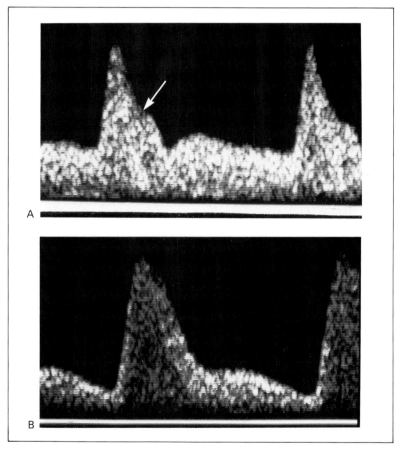

Fig. 13.9 (a) A waveform from a pathological uteroplacental circulation. (b) A waveform from the internal iliac artery. Note that the pathological uteroplacental waveform has an obvious biphasic systolic deceleration slope (arrow).

c. *Mixed resistance pattern* — one side (usually the placental side) has an RI < 0.58 and the other side has an RI > 0.58.

Problems

1. Inability to acquire any waveforms:
a. Audible but not visualised — check the machine settings as detailed on page 227.
b. No signal; maternal weight more than 140 kg. Give up and consider sending the woman to a centre that has colour coded, pulsed wave Doppler equipment.
c. No signal; correct machine settings. Keeping the Doppler probe upright, place it in the lower, outer quadrant of the uterus close to the midline. Then slowly slide the probe towards the pelvic side wall until either you obtain a signal or are no longer over the uterus. If the probe is no longer over the uterus, point it medially until a signal is obtained from within the uterus (usually the umbilical artery) and then angle the probe laterally until you acquire a signal. If the signal is from the internal iliac artery (Fig. 13.9b) then gently angle the probe more medially and inferiorly.
2. Difficulty in distinguishing waveforms from the internal iliac artery from pathological uteroplacental waveforms. Examine Figures 13.9a & b. The pathological uteroplacental waveforms (Fig. 13.9a) have a biphasic deceleration slope in systole whereas those from the internal iliac artery have a smooth, steep slope.
3. Difficulty in determining if a waveform with a very low RI is from the uteroplacental circulation or from an intervillus space. Only very rarely is the RI from the uteroplacental circulation less than 0.25.

Indication for, and interpretation of uteroplacental waveforms

Currently the following statements are supported by at least one published study:

1. In hypertensive disease of pregnancy the presence of a low resistance pattern is associated with a very low chance of complications. Suggested complication rates are:
a. A less than 5% chance of developing proteinuric hypertension
b. A less than 1% chance of a co-existing small-for-gestational-age fetus
c. An almost zero chance of the hypertensive disease fulminating to produce eclampsia.
2. In hypertensive disease of pregnancy with a high resistance pattern it is very likely that the hypertension is placental in origin and that preterm delivery will be required. In about 50% of cases the reason for early delivery is fulminating proteinuric hypertension and in the remainder the reason is usually a coexisting small-for-gestational-age

fetus that demonstrates absent end-diastolic frequencies in the umbilical artery.

3. In hypertensive disease with a mixed waveform pattern, complication rates are approximately:

a. A 15% incidence of proteinuric hypertension

b. A 50% incidence of co-existent asymmetrically small-for-gestational-age fetuses

c. A less than 5% chance of developing fulminating hypertension.

COMBINED UTEROPLACENTAL AND UMBILICAL ARTERY WAVEFORMS

As the state of the fetal circulation is largely determined by the perfusion of the intervillus space, it is logical to study both circulations in women who present with a real-time diagnosis of a small-for-gestational-age fetus, hypertension or oligohydramnios. Waveforms are acquired as described above and interpreted as follows.

Low resistance uteroplacental waveforms
Normal umbilical artery waveforms

This indicates normal physiological adaptation to pregnancy. Unless the maternal blood pressure needs to be treated with oral antihypertensive agents the woman can be managed as an outpatient with weekly measurements of the umbilical artery if the fetus is asymmetrically small on real-time ultrasound. Fortnightly real-time measurements of growth should also be performed.

Low resistance uteroplacental waveforms
Umbilical artery waveforms with absent end-diastolic frequencies

This indicates that impaired fetal growth is probably due to a primary fetal reason. It is an extremely rare finding (less than 2% of fetuses shown to be small on real-time ultrasound). The fetus should undergo a detailed study of its anatomy to exclude structural anomalies and markers suggestive of chromosomal abnormality (Appendix 3). It is reasonable to perform a cordocentesis in order to karyotype the fetus, to look for TORCH infections and *Listeria*, and to perform blood gases. If these are all normal and the fetus is more than 28 weeks gestation it is probable that the fetus should be delivered. If it is less than 28 weeks gestation it should be referred for detailed examination of the fetal circulation.

High resistance uteroplacental waveforms
Normal umbilical artery waveforms

In this situation the hypertensive aspect of the disease predominates but the fetus rarely suffers except in cases of placental abruption. Half of these women will need a preterm delivery for fulminating hypertension but if the pregnancy continues for long enough then the fetal circulation will also become disturbed.

High resistance uteroplacental waveforms
Absent end-diastolic frequencies in the umbilical artery waveforms

In this situation there is commonly both proteinuric hypertension and asymmetrical intrauterine growth retardation. If the woman is more than 28 weeks gestation then the fetus should be delivered. If she is less than 28 weeks gestation then detailed studies of the fetal circulation are needed (see below).

Mixed resistance pattern in the uteroplacental waveforms
Normal umbilical artery waveforms

There may be a need to control the maternal hypertension with oral agents; if not, the woman can usually be allowed home and the umbilical waveforms can be repeated on a weekly basis.

Mixed resistance pattern in the uteroplacental waveforms
Absent end-diastolic frequencies in the umbilical artery waveforms

In this situation the intrauterine aspects of reduced placental perfusion predominate and the fetus should be delivered if it is more than 28 weeks gestation. If it is less, detailed studies of the fetal circulation are required.

In the presence of **oligohydramnios** the combination of waveforms can be interpreted as follows.

High resistance uteroplacental waveforms
Absent end-diastolic frequencies in the umbilical artery waveforms

Diagnosis: Placental insufficiency
Prognosis: Intrauterine death (90%)
Management: Check for the presence of the lupus anticoagulant (which can be treated with aspirin and steroids). Give low dose aspirin, which maintains the uteroplacental circulation in its current state rather than allowing further deterioration. Follow-up should be by weekly Doppler ultrasound of the umbilical circulation and fortnightly growth scans.

Low resistance uteroplacental waveforms
Absent end-diastolic frequencies in the umbilical artery waveforms

Diagnosis: Primary fetal cause
Management: Detailed ultrasound examination looking for structural
abnormalities, cordocentesis for karyotyping and a search for
intrauterine infections.

High resistance uteroplacental waveforms
Normal umbilical artery waveforms

Diagnosis: Placental insufficiency
Management: If there has been severe oligohydramnios (no pool
greater than 1 cm depth) over the period of 16–22 weeks gestation it is
very likely that the baby will die from pulmonary hypoplasia if it
survives to term. Treatment with low dose aspirin may improve fetal
growth but we are unsure if it will improve survival.

Low resistance uteroplacental waveforms
Normal umbilical artery waveforms

Diagnosis: The most likely cause is rupture of the fetal membranes.
This may be confirmed by the instillation of very dilute methylene blue
via amniocentesis. The prognosis is poor if the membranes have
ruptured before 22 weeks gestation. In the absence of infection the
outlook is much better for rupture of the membranes at later gestations.

COLOUR CODED AND PULSED DOPPLER STUDIES

Currently, virtually all aspects of the use of colour coded or pulsed
Doppler are in the realms of research but they are beginning to be
introduced into patient management in the following circumstances:

*1. For detailed evaluation of the fetal circulation when absence of
end-diastolic frequencies has been demonstrated in the umbilical artery but
delivery is not considered desirable because of prematurity.* Chronic
underperfusion of the intervillus space (placental insufficiency) is
probably always due to abnormal invasion by the placenta into the
maternal spiral arteries. This usually results in a high resistance or a
mixed resistance pattern in the uteroplacental circulation. The
decreased perfusion causes spasm and then occlusion of the resistance
vessels on the fetal side of the placenta (the tertiary stem arterioles).
The increased resistance causes blood returning to the placenta to be
shunted to the fetal brain, coronary arteries and adrenal glands and
leads to asymmetrical intrauterine growth retardation. Initially these
changes are to the fetus's benefit as oxygenated blood is presented first

to the fetal brain. If these changes are prolonged then ischaemia may cause renal damage resulting in oligohydramnios, damage to the fetal liver resulting in coagulation problems and damage to the bowel causing necrotising enterocolitis. Eventually, as the placental resistance is increased, the shunting to the fetal brain is reversed and the fetus will die.

Absence of end-diastolic frequencies in the umbilical artery indicates that the shunting has occurred but there appear to be no further consistently recognisable changes in the umbilical circulation prior to the development of an abnormal cardiotocograph and subsequent fetal death. Colour coded Doppler ultrasound allows the easy recognition of the descending fetal aorta and cerebral vessels (many of which are below the resolution of real-time ultrasound) such that the time gate (Ch. 16) of the pulsed, Doppler equipment can be placed over the vessel and a signal obtained. It is now also possible to obtain signals from the renal artery (Fig. 13.10) and the future will probably hold detailed mapping of all major fetal vessels. Currently the waveforms from the descending aorta (Fig. 13.11) and the common carotid (or middle cerebral) artery (Fig. 13.12) are used to determine the degree of shunting.

Figure 13.13 illustrates the ratio of the pulsatility index (PI) from the middle cerebral artery to the descending aorta. Fetuses that have an increasing ratio will probably not die within the next 24 hours whereas those with a decreasing ratio are very likely to die.

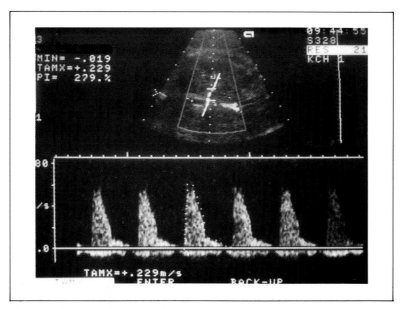

Fig. 13.10 A colour coded Doppler image demonstrating the fetal renal artery.

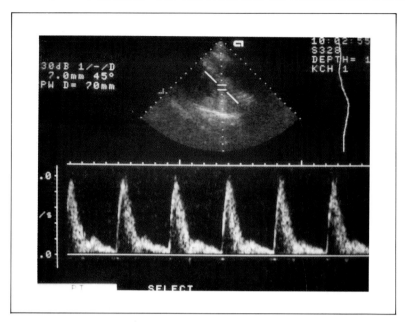

Fig. 13.11 The waveform from the descending fetal aorta.

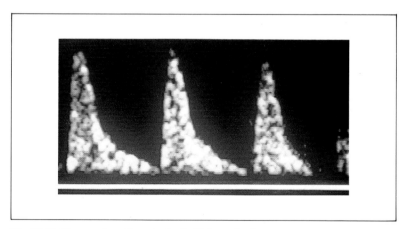

Fig. 13.12 The waveform from the fetal middle cerebral artery.

A dilemma arises because, at presentation, it is impossible to tell whether the ratio is increasing or decreasing so a cordocentesis to measure blood gases (and to determine karyotype) is necessary. If the fetus is both hypoxic and acidotic it should be delivered immediately if it has any chance at all of extrauterine survival (i.e. if it is over 24 weeks gestation and has an estimated weight of more than 450 g). If it is

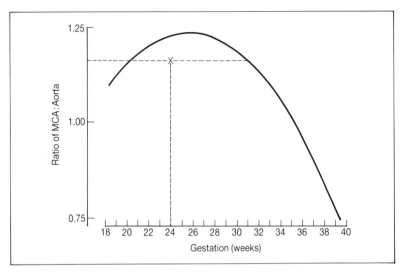

Fig. 13.13 The ratio of the pulsatility indices from the middle cerebral artery (MCA) to the descending aorta. The dotted line indicates a value obtained from a small-for-gestational-age fetus at 24 weeks. As it is a single reading, a cordocentesis is indicated to determine the acid–base status and the degree of hypoxia. If these fall within the normal ranges the fetus can then continue to be monitored by serial determination of the MCA:aorta ratio. A fall in the ratio indicates impending death.

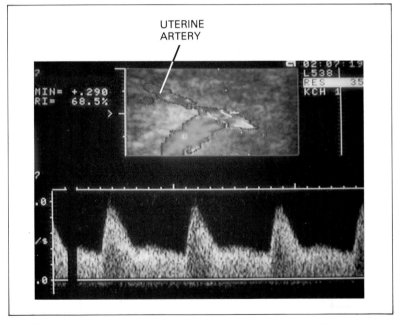

Fig. 13.14 A colour coded, pulsed Doppler image of the uterine artery. The upper panel is a real-time image of the internal iliac artery (blue) and the uterine artery (red). The time gate of the pulsed Doppler is represented by the two short, white lines. The lower panel shows the resultant uterine artery waveform.

normoxic then its progress should be monitored twice daily with pulsed Doppler ultrasound.

2. *To accurately determine the origin of waveforms from the uteroplacental circulation.* It is impossible to determine the precise site of origin of uteroplacental waveforms acquired by means of continuous wave equipment. Although uteroplacental waveforms have vastly improved the prediction of pregnancy outcome in women with hypertension, there is still a false positive rate which some authors believe would be removed if we could ensure that the signal arose from the uterine artery. Figure 13.14 illustrates the use of colour coded, pulsed Doppler equipment to obtain waveforms from the uterine artery. We do not yet know if this will prove to be sufficiently superior to continuous wave equipment to warrant its extra cost.

CHAPTER FOURTEEN
The ultrasound department

We hope that we have demonstrated in the preceding chapters of this book that all women should have at least one ultrasound examination during pregnancy. This chapter is aimed at helping you to provide a routine service.

The requirements in terms of machines and personnel will vary with:

- The number of deliveries per year
- Whether the service is largely routine or is to include 'high risk' referral clinics
- The size of the gynaecological workload.

The following calculations are based upon one ultrasonographer scanning for five days a week with a working year of 46 weeks. We recommend that the minimum time between appointments should be 15 minutes. This will allow 30 women to be scanned in a seven and a half hour day, totalling 6900 scans per year. If the appointment interval is 20 minutes then this reduces the number of women scanned per day to 22 and the annual total to 5060.

Three regimens of routine ultrasound examination are practised:

1. All women are scanned at or soon after their booking appointment irrespective of menstrual age.

2. Women are scanned at 18–20 weeks gestation. We have already detailed (Ch. 5) the advantages of this regimen over (1), and we feel that this makes the best use of invariably limited resources.

3. In addition to (1) and/or (2) a further scan may be performed in the third trimester as a screening test for intrauterine growth retardation (see Ch. 11).

If it is aimed to perform the routine ultrasound examination at 18–24 weeks gestation, a certain number of repeat examinations will be inevitable. As examination of fetal anatomy is best performed during this time we believe that women who have been scanned in early pregnancy should be rescanned at 18–24 weeks gestation. The earlier scan may have been necessary for uncertain menstrual dates, a discrepancy between clinical size and menstrual dates, or a problem of early pregnancy. Women who book after 24 weeks will usually require at least two scans to establish/confirm gestational age (see Ch. 5). Finally, about 10% of women will need to be rescanned because fetal position or maternal obesity makes measurement and examination impossible at this gestation. From the above we estimate that 1300 scans would need to be performed for every 1000 deliveries.

Additional scanning appointments will be necessary for the following problems of later pregnancy:

- Serial scans on 'high risk' women (see Chs 11 and 12)
- Scans to refute or confirm the clinical suspicion of small-for-gestational-age
- Repeat examinations on women with low-lying placentae at the early scan (this is about 5% of the total population)
- Women with clinical suspicion of placenta praevia
- Women needing fetal weight estimates (see Ch. 12)
- Scans for fetal presentation (hopefully not many)
- Urgent scans, e.g. women with preterm labour, suspected IUDs.

This will add approximately a further 300 scans to every 1000 deliveries depending upon the number of 'high risk' women in the population and the skill of the clinicians. Thus for every 1000 deliveries approximately 1600 appointments will be needed.

If a routine scan is performed in the third trimester this will mean a minimum of 2300 scans for every 1000 deliveries. This should reduce the requests for scans to confirm a clinical suspicion of IUGR and placental localisation but will not affect the other requests. This will give a total of approximately 2450 appointments per 1000 deliveries.

As an example, if the delivery rate is 3000 per year then a minimum of 4800 appointments would be needed in order to offer a routine 18–24 weeks examination and further scans as requested by the clinicians. This workload could, in theory, be covered by one full-time ultrasonographer working with a 20 minute appointment system.

Staff turnover is likely to be high if one ultrasonographer is expected to scan at this rate continuously. The quality of the ultrasound examination is very much influenced by the attitude as well as the skill of the ultrasonographer. Once the scanning load is seen as boring, repetitive and unrewarding, the accuracy of measurements and the thoroughness of every examination will suffer.

Ultrasound examinations are performed best if they can be seen to be an important part of the woman's management. This depends upon the relationship and understanding between the obstetric and ultrasound departments. Ideally, the ultrasound department should be under the control and supervision of an obstetric ultrasonographer. This means that he/she is available to give an immediate opinion on suspect ultrasound findings and can assess their relevance to patient management.

If the ultrasound department is not run by an obstetrician or a radiologist with a real interest in obstetric ultrasound it is often difficult to influence the clinicians to make optimum use of the facilities available. As the clinician is finally responsible for the woman's welfare the rule must be 'scan first and argue later'. Carefully worded reports with sensible suggestions as to the interpretation of the findings and the timing of a re-examination (if appropriate) are often the first steps in establishing a working relationship.

Anomalies or severe growth retardation should be communicated by telephone to the clinician responsible for the woman's care. It is not good enough to send the woman away and send a written report in due course.

PRACTICAL ASPECTS IN THE RUNNING OF A DEPARTMENT

The structure of an ultrasound department

Location

Ideally, it should be situated close to the antenatal department but should not be within the antenatal clinic or wards. The ultrasound department runs best if the administration is separate from that of the antenatal clinic and this is encouraged by having a separate department.

Space

We suggest the following as the minimum of space requirements for the ultrasound department.

1. A separate room for each ultrasound machine to include:
   (i) The machine and the operator's stool
   (ii) The examination couch, with a tilting foot. Steps should be provided to allow the pregnant woman to climb onto the couch.
   (iii) Space for the partner and a pushchair
   (iv) Space for the woman's belongings
   (v) A desk on which to write reports.
2. A reception and filing area to include:
   (i) A receptionist's desk, chair and telephone
   (ii) Filing cabinets to store ultrasound records for all currently pregnant women.
3. A waiting area for up to four women per machine. There should also be space for partners, children, pushchairs and shopping. If

this area is close to the reception area it should be large enough to accommodate women waiting to make appointments.

4. Changing cubicles. These may not be strictly necessary but should be available if possible. There should be two per machine and each should contain a chair and hanging facilities for the women's clothes. They should be warm.
5. Toilets and washing facilities. Ideally, there should be separate facilities for staff and patients.
6. Storage space. This should be large enough to store acoustic oil, hard copy, patients' gowns, bed linen and paper, stationery, and as many years' worth of old records as the department wishes to keep (see also Legal requirements).
7. A small refrigerator (4°C).
8. A supply of anti-D gammaglobulin.
9. A staff room or at the very least lockers for staff belongings.
10. Ideally, a room somewhat removed from the main department in which parents can be counselled. This should have a separate telephone so that calls can be made to referring consultants in private.
11. There should be a ready supply of drinking water for those women whose bladders need filling.

Staffing the department

The ultrasonographers. The number of these will depend upon the workload, and guidelines are given earlier in the chapter.

The receptionist. If the department is to run efficiently then the ultrasonographers are best employed performing examinations and interpreting the results, not answering the telephone, making appointments and showing patients where to change. These functions and the filing of reports are best done by a receptionist.

Nurses/midwives. If there are no medical or midwifery ultrasonographers in the department, nursing or medical cover should be easily available if emergencies arise. If the department also carries out invasive procedures under ultrasound control then nursing assistance may also be needed to cover these sessions. Male ultrasonographers may also require a nurse when employing vaginal ultrasound.

Running costs

The ultrasound service, once set up, is very cheap to run compared with other imaging services. The initial outlay will include the ultrasound machines, the departmental furniture including the examination couches, gestation calculators and electronic calculators, video equipment and cameras.

Running costs should include:

- A servicing contract for each machine. This can be obtained from most manufacturers but may be unnecessary if the hospital medical physics department is prepared to provide maintenance
- A means of making hard copy
- Acoustic oil
- Paper towels, couch rolls, stationery
- Laundry for bed linen, patients' gowns and staff uniforms
- Cleaning.

Writing reports

The aim of the ultrasound report is to communicate the findings to the clinician as clearly as possible. There is no doubt that size and growth is best recorded by graphical means. We suggest the following:

1. The person performing the ultrasound examination should always fill in the chart, write the report and interpret the findings.
2. Charts should be used that are easy to understand and that can be securely inserted into the woman's notes.
3. Although the graphic presentation is easy to understand, there should be space for recording measurements and for the ultrasonographer to make comments on the interpretation of the ultrasound findings.
4. The charts should be available each time the woman attends for examination so that they may be updated. Issuing new charts at each visit will guarantee that the most important findings are overlooked.
5. The following must be included on the charts:
   a. The woman's name and hospital number
   b. The date of the ultrasound examination
   c. The ultrasound measurements and findings
   d. Interpretation of ultrasound measurements. If the ultrasound prediction of the delivery date is different to that from the menstrual dates this should be clearly stated (see Ch. 5). We suggest that having once established gestational age by ultrasound, all subsequent measurements are plotted according to the ultrasound assigned EDD. Plotting measurements according to both ultrasound and postmenstrual age is confusing and unnecessary.
   e. The ultrasonographer's signature.
6. The interpretation of ultrasound findings and therefore the decision to rescan should rest largely with the ultrasonographer. Appointments for further examinations should be made at the time of the initial examination so that they are not overlooked in the administration of the antenatal clinic. In this way the department

will best serve its pregnant population but if there are clinical indications for a re-examination at a different time these must obviously be accommodated.

7. Ultrasound reports should be legible and as succinct as possible.

What records to keep

There is no agreed policy as to which measurements and images should be recorded. We suggest the following:

1. In an apparently normal pregnancy

a. *18–24 week scan.* Hard copy that contains the woman's name and which demonstrates the sections from which the relevant measurements were taken. This is usually a Polaroid picture or a thermal image. In addition, a record of which organ systems have been examined should be kept. This is best performed by ticking a checklist. The position of the placenta and the amount of amniotic fluid should also be noted.

b. *32–36 week scan.* The minimum that is necessary at this time is a record of the section on which the AC was measured and a comment on the amount of amniotic fluid and the position of the placenta.

2. In an abnormal pregnancy

a. *Suspected fetal abnormality.* The entire examination is best recorded on videotape as this allows easy review by obstetricians, paediatricians, paediatric surgeons and geneticists as well as a chance to demonstrate the abnormality to the parents. Failing this, multiple still images should be taken.

b. *Abnormalities of growth.* Relevant sections on which the growth parameters have been measured should be kept together with some comment on the amount of amniotic fluid.

Doppler waveforms. Hard copy of representative waveforms should be stored in the women's notes.

Legal requirements

1. All records relating to a pregnancy must be kept for 17 years.

2. The person signing the report is responsible for the accuracy of the measurements and the plots. The final responsibility for the interpretation of the results rests with the clinician.

3. *Missed abnormalities.* There are little or no guidelines on the responsibility of the ultrasonographer for detecting abnormalities. On general principles you would probably be held responsible for overlooking the following:

— Multiple pregnancy
— Placenta praevia
— Gross abnormalities such as anencephaly.

— Large masses or cysts within or attached to the fetus, e.g. cystic hygroma, omphalocoele.
— Obvious disparities between limb lengths and head and body size. For example, a small BPD and HC compared to appropriate limb and AC measurements may indicate the presence of spina bifida.

You should also be aware of abnormalities that may present later in pregnancy and take the appropriate precautions after discussion with the clinician. For example, women at risk of microcephaly should be offered serial ultrasound examinations.

Abnormalities of the kidneys, heart and late deviations from normal growth are more likely to be missed either because they present as relatively subtle changes or because they were not present at the time of the routine ultrasound.

CHAPTER FIFTEEN
Basic physics and ultrasound machines

INTRODUCTION

The use of ultrasound for medically diagnostic purposes was developed from SONAR (Sound Navigation And Ranging) systems used to detect submarines. In order to attempt to understand how ultrasound is used to display images it is necessary to be aware of some sound wave theory, much of which can be understood without the need for complex mathematical formulae.

SOME SOUND WAVE THEORY

Definitions

Sound is the orderly transmission of mechanical vibrations through a medium; disorderly vibrations are known as *noise*. In order for these vibrations to be propagated a physical medium is needed. Such media are composed of particles, and the sound vibrations travel through the medium by a series of compression and then rarefaction of the particles (Fig. 15.1a).

Most commonly the particles oscillate in the direction of propagation of the wave (longitudinal wave). Plotting these oscillations against time usually produces a sine wave (Fig. 15.1b). The *amplitude* (A) of a waveform is the height of the apex above the baseline whilst the *wavelength* (λ) is the distance between two consecutive, equivalent points on the waveform.

The number of vibrations that occur per second is known as the *frequency* and is measured in hertz (Hz), 1 Hz being 1 cycle/s. The human ear can detect frequencies in the range of 20 Hz to 20 kilohertz (20 000 Hz). Sound above this range is known as ultrasound; most instruments used in diagnostic medicine function in the range of 1–10 megahertz (MHz), 1 MHz being 1 000 000 cycles/s.

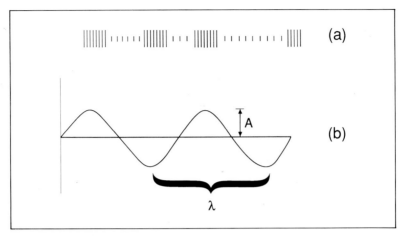

Fig. 15.1 (a) Compression and rarefaction of air particles that allow sound to travel through air. (b) A sine wave showing oscillations against time (A = amplitude, λ = wavelength).

Sound velocity

In order to produce sound (or ultrasound) a device which will vibrate in sympathy to an electrical signal is needed. Examples of familiar devices are tuning forks and loudspeakers. Ultrasound is generated from crystals that demonstrate the piezoelectric property. When electrical pulses are applied across the face of such crystals the thickness of the crystal changes causing it to vibrate, transmitting compression waves into the human body. Piezoelectric crystals can also act as ultrasound receivers in that any pressure waves that they receive are converted into electrical signals. Quartz crystals are sometimes used but most modern ultrasound crystals use thin plates or discs of ceramic which are silver plated to form the electrical connections. The ceramic material and dimensions determine the frequency of operation with the higher operating frequencies resulting from the thinner and smaller crystals.

The speed of propagation of sound through a medium is determined by mechanical properties such as density and elasticity (compliance). Thus bone, which is both dense and compliant, has a sound velocity in the range of 2700–4000 m/s, whereas lung tissue, which is light and non-compliant, has a sound velocity of 650–1160 m/s. The human body is mostly composed of water, which has a sound velocity of approximately 1500 m/s.

The depth of a structure within the body can be determined if the velocity of ultrasound is known, and the time taken for the ultrasound beam to travel to the structure and back (go–return time) can be measured:

Depth = 2 × velocity/go–return time

Velocity (c) affects the frequency (f) and wavelength (λ) of ultrasound as follows:

$$\lambda = c/f$$

As the velocity of ultrasound in a given medium is constant, the wavelength and frequency have an inverse relationship.

Sound attenuation

As ultrasound travels into a medium its energy is absorbed by the particles in that medium. This results in a decrease in amplitude that is exponential to the distance travelled. This decrease is known as attenuation and is expressed in decibels per centimetre (dB/cm); it is constant for a given medium at a given frequency. Table 15.1 lists the ultrasonic properties of some common media. In soft tissue the attenuation is assumed to be 1 dB/cm (at 1 MHz) so that a 5 MHz wave attenuates at 5 dB/cm. In air, however, the attenuation coefficient is dependent upon the square of the frequency so that a 5 MHz wave will attenuate at 25 dB/cm, making air a poor transmitting medium for ultrasound.

Table 15.1 Ultrasonic properties of common media

Medium	Propagation velocity (m/s)	Attenuation coefficient at 1 MHz (dB/cm)
Air	330	10
Bone	2700–4100	3–10
Fat	1500	1
Lung	650–1160	40
Muscle	1545–1630	1.5–2.5
Soft tissues	1460–1615	0.3–1.5

Decibel notation

In order to compare the change in wave amplitude or intensity, the ratio of the signals is expressed as a logarithm. This removes the need for absolute measurement and provides a simple method for expressing numbers that extend over several decibel orders of magnitude. Moreover, the product of two ratios is obtained simply by summing the decibel value instead of calculations involving ratios. Thus two different intensities, I_1 and I_2 can be expressed in decibels as:

$$dB = 10 \log (I_1/I_2)$$

a positive dB value indicating that I_1 is greater than I_2 and a negative value that I_1 is smaller than I_2.

Table 15.2 Decibel values

Multiplication or division ratio	dB value
1	0
1.25	1
2	3
2.5	4
3	5
5	7
7	8
10	10
100	20
1000	30

Table 15.2 gives the decibel values for numbers up to 1000. Any ratio can be quickly converted into its decibel value by factorising the ratio and summing the dB values of the factors, as in the following two examples:

Ratio: 4
   Factors: 2×2
   dB value $= 3 + 3 = 6\,dB$

Ratio: 350
   Factors: $5 \times 7 \times 10$
   dB $= 7 + 8 + 10 = 25\,dB$

Conversion of dB to the ratio is just as easy:

$22\,dB = 20 + 1 + 1$
Ratio $= 100 + 1.25 + 1.25 = 102.50$

Echoes

Reflection and refraction

Ultrasound travels in straight lines until it meets an interface. An *interface* is defined as a boundary between two tissues which have differing acoustic velocities. When a wave meets an interface a part of the wave is reflected from the interface and the remainder is propagated through the second medium. If the incidence wave meets the interface orthogonally (i.e. at 90°) then the wave will be propagated without deviation into the second medium, and any reflected waves return along the path of the incidental wave. If the wave meets the interface obliquely then the transmitted wave undergoes *refraction* (Fig. 15.2). The degree of refraction and the amplitude of reflection is dependent upon the differences in the sound velocities of the two media. The greater the difference in velocities the greater the amplitude of the

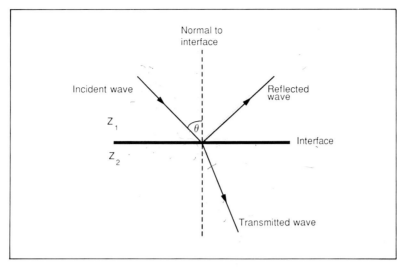

Fig. 15.2 Interaction of a sound wave at an interface. The transmitted wave has undergone refraction (Z_1 and Z_2 are tissues of differing acoustic impedance).

reflected wave and the degree of refraction. Thus the biggest echoes occur when the incident beam is orthogonal to the structure being insonated and the acoustic mismatch at the interface is large, such as occurs at the interface between the soft tissue and the fetal skull. Although the fetal skull causes a large reflection, the energy of the transmitted beam is greatly reduced making deeper structures difficult to image. At gas–soft tissue interfaces the acoustic mismatch is so great that almost all the beam is reflected so that scanning through lung or bowel is impossible.

Scattering

Reflection only occurs when the surface of the interface is smooth and the dimensions are greater than the wavelength of the incidence beam. In the human body, interfaces are rarely smooth so most echoes are produced by scattering. As a guide, reflected echoes contain about 1% of the incident energy whilst scattered echoes contain approximately 0.001%. Fortunately, modern equipment is able to detect such small echoes.

Reverberation

This artifact is illustrated in Figures 15.3 and 15.14 and is responsible for obscuring detail in the proximal part of an image. It occurs when there is a large acoustic mismatch between two media but little attenuation in the first transmitting media.

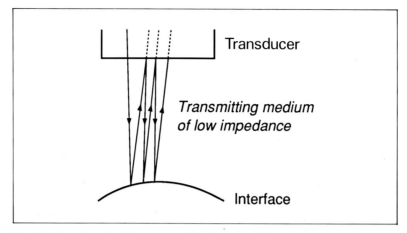

Fig. 15.3 Reverberation. Waves are readily reflected back from the interface as there is little impedance in the transmitting medium. This gives the appearances shown in Fig. 15.14.

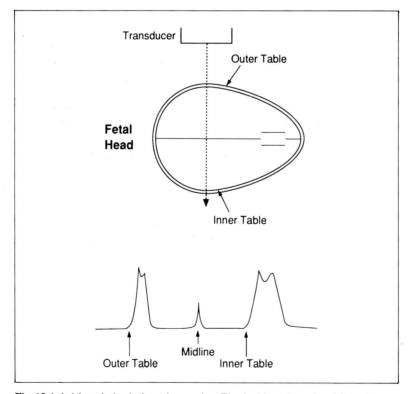

Fig. 15.4 Axial resolution in A-mode scanning. The double peak produced from the parietal bones of the skull indicates that the system is not able to resolve the outer and inner tables of each bone as separate echoes.

ULTRASOUND TRANSDUCERS

Resolution

Resolution is defined as the ability of the system to discriminate adjacent structures. It is divided into:

- Axial resolution
- Lateral resolution.

Axial resolution

This is the ability to distinguish between structures that lie in line with the ultrasound beam (Fig. 15.4). The features of a transducer that determine axial resolution are dampening (ringdown) and wavelength.

Ringdown

When a piezoelectric crystal is rung by means of an electronic pulse the vibrations must be dampened before the crystal can receive returning echoes. The time taken to perform this is known as the ringdown time.

Ringdown is measured in cycles and is counted by the number of half cycles needed for the oscillations of the piezoelectric crystal to decay to 10% of the maximum peak-to-peak amplitude (-20 dB). One half cycle is added and the number is divided by two; for example, if five half cycles are required for the vibrations to decay to 10% of maximum then ringdown equals three cycles. Measuring ringdown time also allows determination of spatial pulse length, which is the actual physical space occupied by the burst of ultrasound. Figure 15.5 shows a simple time–rate–distance relationship for an ultrasonic wave. In this example, by the time the vibrations have been dampened to -20 dB, the

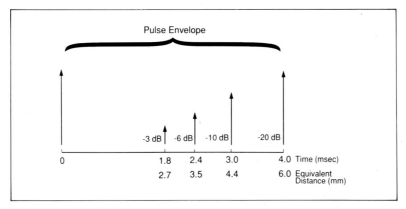

Fig. 15.5 Time–rate–distance relationship for an ultrasound wave — used to measure ringdown.

ultrasonic wavefront has travelled 6 mm, i.e. the spatial pulse length is 6 mm. This means that the first 6 mm of tissue cannot be visualised, but also limits resolution of reflecting structures to 6 mm. In practice, ringdown time has to be a compromise between limiting ringing to improve axial resolution and allowing the crystal to ring sufficiently long enough to provide adequate acoustic energy for penetration and echo formation.

Frequency

The frequency of the transducer determines not only axial and lateral resolution (see below) but also the depth to which the ultrasound beam can penetrate. If all other factors are held constant, increasing the ultrasound frequency increases the axial resolution but unfortunately the depth of penetration is reduced because of attenuation. In soft tissue:

Attenuation = 1 dB/cm/MHz × frequency

When imaging superficial structures such as the thyroid gland, a higher frequency transducer (usually 7 MHz) can be used. With a deeper structure, such as a kidney or fetus, greater penetration is needed and a lower frequency transducer such as 3.5 MHz has to be used.

Lateral resolution

This is defined as the ability to distinguish between reflecting surfaces that lie at right angles to the ultrasound beam. If the beam is narrow enough to pass between both reflectors then they can be resolved; hence beam width is the major determinant of lateral resolution.

When a short pulse of ultrasound is transmitted, a broad band of frequencies is generated, known as the *frequency bandwidth*. The frequency ascribed to the transducer is the central frequency of the bandwidth. The *beam width* is defined as the diameter of the ultrasound beam at a standard reference point along its length. The beam width, and therefore lateral resolution, is dependent upon the geometry of the crystal, the frequency and the focusing elements in front of and behind the crystal.

The geometry of the crystal

Crystals that are circular produce a beam having a cylindrical cross-section in which the lateral resolution is uniform across the entire beam. Rectangular crystals, such as those used in linear array transducers, produce a beam having an elliptical cross-section, and lateral resolution is better across the shorter radius of the beam (Fig. 15.6).

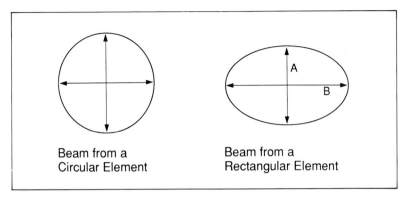

Fig. 15.6 Cross-sections of ultrasound beams. The circular beam has uniform lateral resolution whereas the lateral resolution of the elliptical beam is better in plane A than plane B.

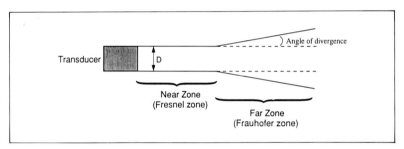

Fig. 15.7 Ultrasound beam demonstrating the near and far zones with the angle of divergence (D = crystal diameter).

Figure 15.7 represents a beam produced by a non-focused, circular crystal. The region where the beam shape is approximately cylindrical is known as the near field (Fresnel zone) and the region of slow divergence is known as the far field (Frauhofer zone). The length of the near field (N) is given by:

$$N = d^2/4\lambda$$

where d is the crystal diameter and λ is the wavelength.

The length of the near field affects the image in the following two ways:

1. The peak acoustic intensity of a transducer occurs at the end of the near field. Non-focused transducers can be used up to approximately twice this distance but thereafter the image deteriorates because the beam diverges.

2. A transducer can only have its maximum acoustic intensity

adjusted or focused at a distance less than or equal to the length of the near field and not to any arbitrary distance further than this.

The divergence that occurs in the far field is given by:

$sin\theta = 1.22 \ \lambda/d$

where θ is the angle of divergence.

As the diameter of the crystal increases, the length of the near field increases and the angle of divergence of the far field decreases; therefore, larger crystals produce narrower beams. Final choice of crystal diameter also depends upon its application, for instance transducers used in paediatric cardiology are limited in size by the need to fit between ribs.

Frequency

Higher frequency beams are less divergent. The explanation can be drawn from Figure 15.7. Since:

$\lambda = c/f$

where λ is the wavelength, c is the propagation velocity, and f is the ultrasound frequency, then the equation for near field length may be re-expressed as:

$N = d^2f/4c$

The formula for far field divergence may be re-expressed as:

$sin \ \theta = 1.22c/f.d$

Increasing the frequency therefore increases the near field length and decreases the angle of far field divergence, once again producing an effectively narrower beam.

Focusing

Focusing a transducer refers to methods of regulating the beam width and of adjusting the region of maximum intensity. Focusing may be carried out by internal or external means. Figure 15.8 illustrates these methods. Internal focusing is achieved by manufacturing a crystal which produces a shallow concave element. The radius of the element, in combination with the frequency and the crystal size, determines the focal point (peak acoustic intensity) of the transducer. A flat epoxy face is then applied over the element. With external focusing a flat crystal is used and a concave acoustic face is applied to the crystal. Internally focused transducers have a flat face which facilitates good patient contact but concave crystals are difficult to manufacture, especially above 5 MHz, because they are too fragile.

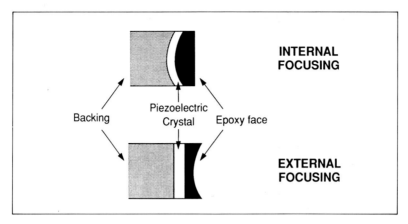

Fig. 15.8 Simple methods of focusing transducers.

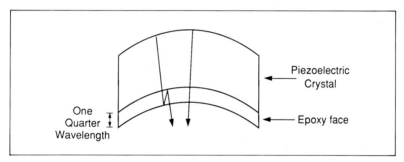

Fig. 15.9 Illustration of the quarter wavelength theory of focusing (see text for explanation).

A further method of focusing relies upon the quarter wavelength focusing theory. Figure 15.9 illustrates such a transducer. The crystal is internally focused and then the epoxy face, which is precisely one-quarter of the transducer wavelength, is applied. Thus an oblique incident wave will be reflected at the epoxy–soft tissue interface and again at the epoxy–crystal interface such that the resulting wave corresponds with the wave that hits the interface at right angles (Fig. 15.9).

Whilst focusing can only adjust the focal point within the near field the *focal zone* may extend into the far field. The focal zone is a transducer parameter that indicates the depths at which the transducer is designed to be most effective. The focal zone extends either side of the focal depth (to the depth of maximum intensity). Its limits are usually defined as the two depths where the ultrasound intensity falls to 3 dB (or half the intensity) at the focal depth.

Focusing helps to improve the detail of an ultrasound image because it creates a narrower beam over a defined focal zone. The selection of a focal zone for a transducer depends upon the depth of the tissue of interest. It is designed such that the narrowest part of the beam is in the region under study. Standard obstetric transducers tend to use large crystals of intermediate frequency (3.5 MHz) with a focal zone of 6–13 cm.

By applying two epoxy faces, each one-quarter of the wavelength in thickness, the focusing effect can be increased, which gives the following clinical improvements:

1. *Increased sensitivity.* This allows a choice of: high quality images at lower acoustic powers (see 'Safety of ultrasound'), the use of lower gain settings so that the signal to noise ratio is increased, or increased penetration.

2. *Increased bandwidth.* A single layer transducer tends to act as a frequency filter allowing less frequencies to pass than with non-focused transducers. Multilayered transducers produce a beam with a broader bandwidth because although they still filter frequencies this is less than with a single layered transducer. Broad bandwidths provide short spatial pulse widths therefore assuring excellent axial resolution.

So far, only mechanical means of focusing transducers have been discussed, but focusing can also be achieved by electronic means (see 'Phased array transducers').

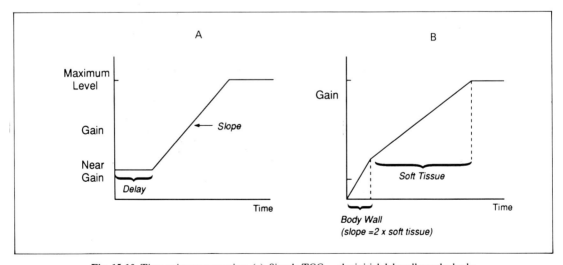

Fig. 15.10 Time-gain compensation. (a) Simple TGC — the initial delay allows the body wall and the full bladder to be ignored whilst the slope reflects the gain applied with time (depth). The curve flattens in the far field as increasing the gain at this depth will only increase machine noise. (b) Complex TGC — this consists of a series of slopes that are tailored for the tissue encountered at various depths; for example, the slope over the body wall is twice that of the soft tissue as muscle has twice the attenuation of soft tissues.

UNWANTED ULTRASOUND EFFECTS

Attenuation and Time — Gain Compensation (TGC)

If two similar interfaces at different depths are insonated they will both produce echoes of similar amplitude but the echo from the deeper interface will be smaller because both the transmitted sound wave and the echo have passed through more tissue and are therefore more attenuated. The deeper the interface and the greater the tissue attenuation the more the received echo must be amplified. This is achieved by TGC, where the receiver amplification (or gain) is increased with increasing time after each transmitted pulse.

Figure 15.10 illustrates a simple TGC. The concept can be extended to allow multiple slopes to compensate for tissues with differing attenuation as in Figure 15.10b.

Noise and other unwanted signals

In general terms any signal other than the desired one could be described as noise. In practice there are two principle sources of unwanted signal:

1. *Other signals*. These are echoes emanating from unwanted ultrasound scattering interfaces which do not contribute to the image quality. They can be overcome by good transducer focusing and by good scanning technique.

2. *Noise*. All electrical components generate white noise, which is random signal occurring across the whole frequency range of the electrical circuits. Noise is also generated by ultrasound scattering in tissue where the speckled effect (for example from liver tissue) contains some random scattering elements. True noise can be distinguished from wanted echoes because the wanted echoes have a predictable characteristic as time passes. Thus, by comparing a real-time image with a previous image, the wanted echoes will occur in the same pattern in both images whereas noise will not. Therefore, if several real-time images are superimposed, the noise can be substantially reduced by electronically eliminating nonrecurring echoes; this technique is known as image correlation. Other techniques, such as filtering, use of thresholds or limiters, may be used to enhance the ratio of signal to noise.

IMAGES

Information from echoes can be displayed in one of four ways:

- Amplitude (A) mode
- Brightness (B) mode

   a. Static images
   b. Real-time images
- Time-motion (T-M) mode
- Doppler ultrasound.

Amplitude (A) mode

In this mode echoes are received by the transducer and converted into voltages, which are displayed as deflections on the y-axis of a cathode ray tube (Fig. 15.4). The height of the deflections corresponds to the amplitude of the echoes, whilst the distance between the echoes represents the distance between the interfaces that produced the echoes.

Brightness (B) mode

Static images

In B-mode scanning the returning echo is converted to a voltage but then displayed on the screen as a bright spot at a position that corresponds to the origin of the echo. The combination of many thousands of such spots, which vary in intensity according to the strength of the echo, will produce a two-dimensional image (Fig. 15.11). In static scanning the transducer is moved manually over the target and the supporting gantry must be able to accurately detect the position of the transducer so that echoes may be accurately plotted in relation to each other.

Real-time images

Real-time images are a rapid series of static images. Their quality depends upon the frame rate, the line density and the field of view. In

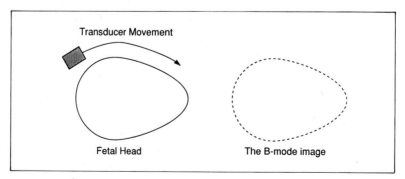

Fig. 15.11 Diagram to illustrate how coalescing echoes form a fetal head in B-mode scanning.

order to keep the image flicker free it must be displayed more than 20 times per second. The acoustic information in each single real-time sweep is therefore much less than in a single sweep, static B-mode scan. For example, a static B-mode scan takes about one second to complete and contains about 500 lines of acoustic information, whereas a single real-time sweep is complete in about 25 milliseconds and contains only 100 lines of information. Additional lines of information may be added electronically by duplicating or averaging adjacent lines but whilst these improve the appearance of the image they do not increase the resolution. Transducer size also limits field of view but increasing the size of the transducer is usually limited by practicalities such as the curvature of the maternal abdomen.

Real-time images can be produced by the following means:

- Mechanical sector transducers
- Electronic linear array transducers
- Electronic phased array transducers.

Mechanical sector transducers. These instruments produce and collect echoes by mechanically rotating three or four crystals about a central axis. As the transducers rotate they are activated in turn and produce a wedge-shaped field of view. The transducers are contained in an oil sealed cylinder and the beam is propagated through the oil, through a plastic window in the housing cylinder and into the patient. The head of the transducer is small in size and so allows scanning into difficult sites, such as the neonatal brain, using the fontanelles as acoustic windows. The main disadvantages are that the apex of the wedge-shaped field of view contains little or no acoustic information and the small transducer size limits the field of view.

A variation on this principle is to use a single transducer crystal and cause it to oscillate back and forth over an angle of 90° or so (this transducer is commonly known as a wobbler).

Linear array transducers. The transducer contains 20–400 separate piezoelectric crystals laid side by side. In order to generate an ultrasound beam the crystals are activated in groups which then effectively behave as a single crystal. This is advantageous in that if the beam was produced by a single large crystal the beam would rapidly diverge (see 'Lateral resolution') whereas the beam produced from the groups of small crystals produces a near field and divergence that are dependent upon the diameter of each crystal. Lateral resolution, therefore, depends upon the ability to generate a well defined beam from a number of crystal elements.

In such apparatus the means of producing rapid scans is by electronically firing adjacent groups of crystals. The crystal elements are usually fired after advancing one crystal element at a time, for example 1 to 7, 2 to 8, 3 to 9 and so on. This produces slightly fewer lines of echo information than the number of crystals in the group.

Furthermore, if the crystals at the edge of the group are activated slightly before those in the centre, this helps to keep the beam parallel to the plane of the scan. This focuses the beam in the x-axis of the transducer (see 'Focusing', under 'Lateral resolution').

The image format in linear array is rectangular with the length corresponding to the depth of visualisation and the width corresponding to the width of the array. By moving the beam electronically (as opposed to mechanically), very high frame rates (up to 70 per second) can be obtained but this is associated with a reduction in line density. Furthermore, high frequency transducers tend to be shorter — for example 3.5 MHz transducers are about 10 cm long by 2 cm wide whereas 5 MHz transducers are about 6 cm long by 1.5 cm wide — reducing the field of view.

Phased array transducers. These transducers also contain lines of crystals that are fired electronically. They are fired in groups as in the linear array transducer but the beam can be steered electronically by altering the timing of the electronic pulses that are applied to each element. A maximum deviation of about 20° is possible.

Focusing is achieved in phased array transducers by use of the wave interference principle. By firing the outer elements of the array before the central ones a curved wavefront is produced, which results in a focal region rather than a focal point. The depth of the focal region can be varied by altering the delays applied to the firing sequence, with one set of delays producing a focal region at a single depth. However, the real-time image may be built up by using a series of pulses for each depth. The first wavefront is arranged to produce echoes from the superficial structures only. A second wavefront is then produced that produces echoes from a deeper layer; a range gate is used to limit the instrument's reception of echoes (see 'Pulsed Doppler flowmeters'). Further depth layers are then acquired one layer at a time, thus giving excellent resolution at all depths of the image.

This technique is also used in linear array transducers. The smaller in size and the greater in number are the crystals, the more effective the focusing and beam steering becomes.

Commonly six depth layers are used. The process is often referred to as *dynamic focusing*. As the deeper levels are imaged the number of elements of the array must be increased but as the sensitivity of the probe increases with its area this also improves resolution. Dynamic focusing increases the ultrasound exposure of the patient (see 'Safety of ultrasound') and it also slows the frame rate. In order to overcome this latter problem many machines allow the operator to single out a single level at which the focusing is optimised.

By applying a delay to returning echoes a single wavefront may be focused at several depths. Echoes take progressively longer to reach the outer elements of the array. Therefore, by delaying the reception of the signal to those elements in the centre of the array, all the returning signals are in phase, thus producing a larger voltage for detection and display. However, signals returning from structures away from the axis of the beam will be even more out of phase with signals in the beam axis and so will be much reduced in amplitude.

These delays in firing the elements of the array and in presenting the echoes are controlled by computer software. This has now reached the stage where electronic focus can allow sharply focused focal zones from the skin to the maximum scanning depth, thus overcoming the limits of resolution imposed by fixed focal point transducers with small crystal diameters.

DISPLAYING IMAGES

Scan converters

A major development in ultrasound imaging was the scan converter, which electronically stored and then produced the scan in a form which could be displayed on a television monitor. For a short time cumbersome analogue scan converters were used, but all modern equipment uses digital storage techniques controlled by a microprocessor. The image consists of a matrix of many thousand picture elements (pixels). The information about the echo amplitude for each pixel is stored as a digital number which relates to the strength of the echo and the resultant intensity of the display. The number of shades of grey is determined by the size of the digital memory elements. Thus a 4 bit system would have 16 different shades of grey (4 bits is $2 \times 2 \times 2 \times 2 = 16$) whereas an 8 bit system would have 256 shades. A typical modern scanner would have a display matrix of 256×256 pixels (a total of 65 000), and each pixel would have an 8 bit number (known as a byte) with 256 possible shades of grey.

Pre-processing

The human eye can only perceive a limited number of shades of grey, especially when displayed on a television screen. Thus the dynamic range of the echo amplitude has to be compressed from 256:1 (or 24 dB) to about 16:1 (or 12 dB). This compression is known as pre-processing and is usually performed in such a way as to prevent the stronger echoes saturating weak echoes, such as those that arise from organ parenchyma. This compression usually means that, in theory, 4 bit digitisers are sufficient for ultrasound machines but rounding errors in division result in loss of signal information so 8 bit processors are used in the most expensive machines.

Post-processing (gamma correction)

Post-processing compensates for nonlinear characteristics of a television monitor as seen by the human eye. For instance, if the signal amplitude of an echo is halved, the perceived intensity of a spot on the television will be much less than half. Thus the amplitude range of 256:1 is altered to produce an image with acceptable levels of greys, whilst at the same time the amplitude range is reduced to the 16:1 dynamic range for television display. This process is known as gamma correction and some machines offer several different corrections ranging from very soft with a maximum number of grey scales to almost bistable for imaging blood vessels.

Zoom

Most scan converters have a zoom facility. This may be a read zoom, in which an area of stored information is selected and then is magnified for display, or it may be a write zoom. In the latter case, the area of interest is selected before storage and then the entire scan converter memory is used to store the data for this region. Write zooms therefore maintain image resolution whereas read zooms do not.

Recent developments

Digital scan converters have few disadvantages, the most significant of which is pixel dropout, where empty pixels in or near images appear as artifacts. This can be overcome by using a computer to vary the size of the pixels. With phased array transducers there are more ultrasound

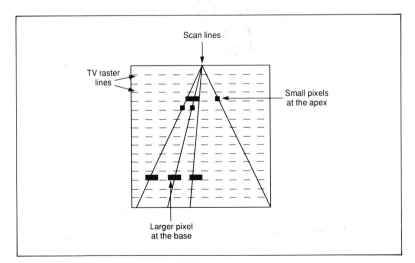

Fig. 15.12 Adaptation of pixel size to fit the space between ultrasound scan lines.

scan lines per unit distance at the apex of the image than at the base. Figure 15.12 demonstrates that this can be overcome by gradually increasing the pixel size, which prevents pixel dropout and gives an effective increase in pixel density. This improves the sharpness of edges of structures and tissue contrast resolution.

TIME-MOTION (T-M) MODE

This mode is used to record fast moving structures such as heart valves, which, if viewed in real-time appear to move in a series of jumps because the limited real-time frame rate (see 'Real-time images', under 'Images'). In this mode the returning echoes are displayed on a long persistence cathode ray tube or stored in a computer memory. Echoes are displayed as a line of dots that sweep across the screen at a constant rate; thus, static structures appear as straight lines, whereas moving structures produce a wavy line indicating that their position is moving with time. The structure in question is usually located with real time and then a cursor known as an M-line is placed over the desired point. The image is produced by using high pulse repetition frequencies, usually in excess of 600 pulses per minute. Figure 15.13 illustrates a T-M trace of the fetal right atrium and aorta, useful for determining atrial and ventricular rates.

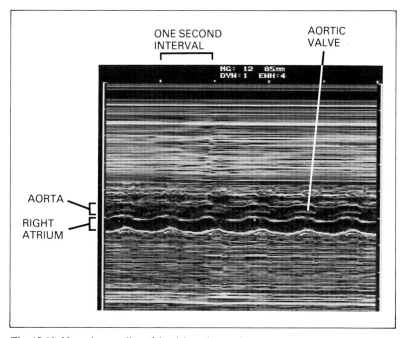

Fig. 15.13 M-mode recording of the right atrium and aorta.

ARTIFACTS

The skill of interpreting real-time images comes from the operator's ability to construct mental three-dimensional images from a series of visualised two-dimensional images. In addition, the operator must be aware of the artifacts that can lead to false interpretations, the most common of which are discussed below.

Refraction

Refraction occurs when the ultrasound beam does not strike the tissue interface orthogonally. It occurs particularly at bone–soft tissue interfaces. The beam may bend as much as 15° and as the echo returns along the same line the operator may be unaware of the bend and therefore misinterprets the true position of the structure. This effect is responsible for many of the misses that occur when tissues are needled under ultrasound guidance.

Reverberation

This occurs when the echo striking the transducer is partially reflected back to the transducer (see 'echoes' above). Reverberation is recognised because it produces a series of regular echoes that decrease in amplitude in regular increments (Figs 15.3 and 15.14). It may be reduced by decreasing the gain or by scanning from a different direction.

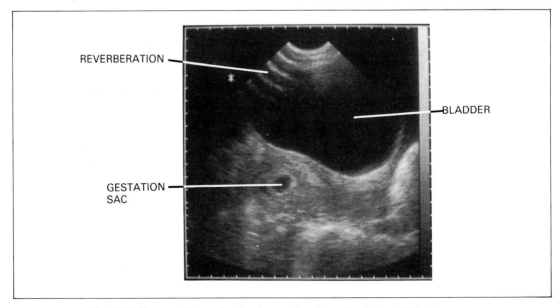

Fig. 15.14 Ultrasound image showing the reverberation artifact in the full bladder.

Side lobe artifacts

These are due to pulses of sound that are generated at the same time as the main pulse but which travel at an angle to the beam. They produce strong echoes that appear as a curved series of bright spots originating from areas with a large impedance gradient such as the interface between the fetal femur and soft tissue. The artifacts can be decreased in size by using more elements in the array and placing them closer together. They can also be reduced by trying to get the structure in question at about 45° to the beam rather than at right angles to it.

CHOICE OF ULTRASOUND MACHINES

Choice of real-time ultrasound machines for obstetrics and gynaecological purposes depends upon the proposed use and the cost. Table 15.3 lists the points to be considered in choosing a machine, but the final decision will often rest with the operator's perception of the image (and cost!).

SAFETY OF ULTRASOUND

Ultrasonic energy is propagated as a pressure wave and the energy crossing a unit per second is called the intensity, which is generally expressed in watts/cm^2. The highest intensities are generated along the beam axis and as the beam spreads out beneath the skin the intensity is reduced. The intensity average across the beam is the spatial averaged (SA) intensity and a measure of the intensity at the beam axis is the spatial peak (SP) intensity.

Diagnostic imaging systems use pulsed ultrasound. Typically real-time ultrasound transducers will emit a pulse 1 microsecond long with a silent period of 1 millisecond during which the sound waves are detected and displayed. This further complication has led to the use of three terms to describe the intensity of an ultrasound wave:

- Temporal average, which is the intensity of sound averaged from one pulse to the next
- Pulse average, which is the intensity measured over the full duration of 1 microsecond of pulsed sound
- Temporal peak, which is the intensity of the maximum amplitude reached within a pulse.

Sound pressure is measured in a water bath using a very small hydrophone. The hydrophone is scanned across and along the beam and a plot is made of the distribution of sound pressure. Beam intensity values are recorded for a particular transducer frequency as spatial peak, temporal average (SPTA) and spatial peak, temporal peak (SPTP).

Table 15.3 Choosing a real-time ultrasound machine

Criteria	Relative importance (0–5)
Image quality	
1. Good resolution from 20–350 mm depth	5
— look for the individual vessels in the cord and the lens in the fetal eye	
2. Low noise and freedom from artifact	4
— look for minimum reverberation in the maternal bladder and little or no grating lobe artifacts	
3. Good textural contrast	5
— Can you clearly distinguish the endometrium from the myometrium? Are the fetal kidneys, liver and lungs clearly distinguished?	
4. Write zoom	3
— Check the detail in the image after zooming	
5. Subjective impression of the image	5
6. If there is an intracavity probe, is the field of view adequate?	4
7. Is the frame rate rapid enough to view moving structures?	4
Technical capabilities	
1. Freeze frame with good image quality	3
2. Interchangeable transducers	2
— As a general rule, buy the machine designed for the intended purpose; machines offering both sector and linear probes are usually a compromise. This, however, is changing with software driven equipment that reconfigures the machine for each probe.	
3. Low ultrasound power output	5
4. Measuring capabilities	2
— Is the precision of the caliper less than 1 mm?	
— Can the control be used with one hand?	3
— Is there an inbuilt delay in circumference measurements to allow easy outlining?	2
— If variable ellipse is the method of measuring circumference/area, is there also a free hand control?	1
— Is there potential for future direct data transfer to computer to avoid transcription errors?	1
— Can errors in circumferences be erased without the need to start again?	1
— Are there inbuilt & appropriate tables?	1
Ergonomics	
1. Is the probe tiring, especially when used in invasive procedures?	4
2. Are biopsy/needle guides available?	2
3. Is the equipment portable (if needed)?	2
Data capture	
1. Can patient identification be put on the screen?	2
2. Is there gamma correction for chosen image mode?	4
3. Is there true video output?	2
4. Hardcopy facility	
— Polaroid	2
— Video printer	5
Finally, will you require 24-hour service and on-site maintenance?	

The mechanisms whereby ultrasound is thought to exert biological effects on tissues may be divided into heat generation and mechanical effects which include cavitation, microstreaming and radiation force. The production of heat is due to absorption of the sound in the medium through which it passes. Experimental evidence has not confirmed any significant temperature rise in mammalian tissue exposed to ultrasound of diagnostic intensities.

Cavitation is caused by oscillation of small gaseous bubbles subjected to pressure waves. These bubbles may then enlarge to a size where they can be maintained (stable cavitation) or they may collapse (transient cavitation). It is probable that the pulses used in diagnostic ultrasound are too short to produce the necessary selective, large amplitude oscillations of microscopic gas bubbles which cause acoustic cavitation. Furthermore, to date no-one has demonstrated that the inert gases required to allow cavitation to occur can be found in the fetus.

Reviewing the positive claims made for ultrasound is difficult. There is no international definition of peak intensity and it is quite probable that the best predictor of transient cavitation is the temporal maximum negative pressure contained in an ultrasound pulse. This information is not available in any published reports.

In the low megahertz frequency range (3–10 MHz) there have been no independently confirmed significant biological effects in mammalian tissues exposed to intensities (SPTA) below 100 mW/cm^2. Furthermore, for ultrasonic exposure times (total time, which includes both off-time and on-time) less than 500 seconds and greater than 1 second, such effects have not been demonstrated even at higher intensities, when the product of intensity and exposure time is less than 50 joules/cm^2.

In order to minimise any potential risk of the relatively high intensities of the duplex, pulsed Doppler systems and colour flow Doppler systems, exposure times should be kept to a minimum. Furthermore, users should ask the manufacturers of their machines to state the levels of ultrasound power output and should then ensure that the lowest power setting is used for measurement. Doppler ultrasound is often quoted as having high power levels but this is not so for all applications because fetal heart rate monitors, for example, employ Doppler ultrasound that operates at very low power levels.

Problems arise when equipment designed for a specific indication is applied to a different situation. For example equipment designed for adult cardiological applications has power levels that are not acceptable for fetal studies. Finally, a distinction must be made between effect and harm. Much of the literature documents a measured effect of ultrasound and infers from this that diagnostic ultrasound may be harmful. However, there is no literature at present which demonstrates such harm from diagnostic ultrasound.

CHAPTER SIXTEEN
The physics of Doppler ultrasound and Doppler equipment

INTRODUCTION

Christian Johann Doppler (1803–1853) described the effect attributed to him by studying light emitted by stars. He observed that light from a star moving away from the earth turned to red whilst that from a star approaching the earth turned to blue. He explained this using some principles of wave theory and started from the assumption that the colour of light varied with its frequency. Doppler postulated that there was a change in the observed colour (frequency) if there was a change in the relative position between the light source and the observer. This shift in the observed frequencies of waves from moving sources is known as the Doppler effect and applies to sound as well as light waves.

THE DOPPLER PRINCIPLE

When a source of sound waves and an observer are approaching each other the observed frequency of the sound is increased. The explanation is that observed frequency of sound depends upon the number of wavefronts reaching the ear per second. The shift between the emitted frequency and the observed frequency is called the Doppler effect. The Doppler shift frequency depends upon the velocity of the source of sound and on the angle from which the direction of movement is observed. This is illustrated in Figure 16.1.

The Doppler shift can be given by the formula:

$f_d = 2f_o \, v/c \, \cos \theta$

where:

f_d is the Doppler shifted frequency
f_o is the frequency of the emitted ultrasound

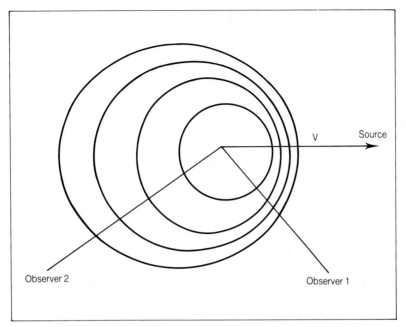

Fig. 16.1 Illustration of the Doppler principle. If a source of sound is moving towards the observer the tone (pitch) of the sound appears to go up as more wavefronts per second reach the observer's ear.

v is the velocity of the moving target

θ is the angle between the ultrasound beam and the direction of movement of the target

c is the propagation of velocity of sound in tissue (assumed to be 1540 m/s).

For example, a 4 MHz Doppler beam which is directly in line with blood moving with a velocity of 1.54 m/s will detect a Doppler shift frequency of:

$$f_d = 2 \times 4 \times 1.54/1540$$
$$= 8/1000 \text{ MHz}$$
$$= 8 \text{ kHz}$$

It follows that the maximum Doppler shift will occur at angles of 0° (maximum positive Doppler shift) and 180° (maximum negative Doppler shift). At an angle of 90° there will be no Doppler shift (cos 90° = 0). Doppler shifted frequencies obtained from flowing blood in the uteroplacental and fetal circulation with angles of insonation of 20–60° are typically in the audible range (up to 12 kHz). This is convenient as it means that the signals may be monitored by loudspeakers and stored on magnetic audio tape for later off-line analysis.

THE DOPPLER FREQUENCY SPECTRUM

It is probable that single blood cells do not produce Doppler echoes as their size is only a fraction of the wavelength of ultrasound. It is more probable that scattering occurs from the random changes in density of blood cells in the plasma. The theory of the production of Doppler shifted frequencies by small targets is complex, but essentially back-scattered echoes from red blood cells are independent of the shape of the target and depend only on its volume and the impedance mismatch of its surroundings. Doppler recorded signals from flowing blood therefore contain a range of frequencies known as the Doppler spectrum. The spectral frequency distribution depends upon the distribution of red blood cell velocities within the blood (the flow velocity profile).

The distribution of velocities of a fluid flowing in a long, straight, smooth sided, non-branching tube is radially symmetrical about the centre of the tube and is defined as laminar flow. Figure 16.2 represents the change in flow velocity profiles as the velocity of the fluid increases. This change in distribution from plug to parabolic flow profiles with increasing velocity is caused mainly by fluid viscosity and friction at the vessel wall. When flow is parabolic the mean velocity is equal to half the maximum velocity whilst for plug velocity profiles the mean velocity is equal to the maximum velocity. Between these two extremes, however, intermediate flow profiles exist so that mean velocity will be between half maximum and maximum velocity.

In the fetal circulation, the descending aorta normally demonstrates

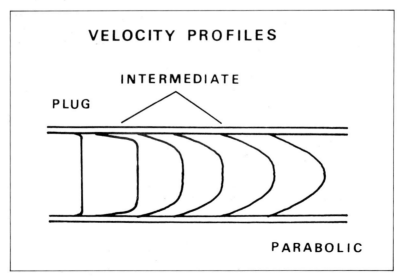

Fig. 16.2 Flow velocity profiles (see text for explanation).

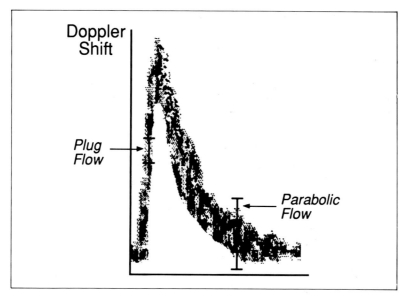

Fig. 16.3 Doppler sonogram from the fetal descending aorta. Note how all the Doppler shifted frequencies are clustered close to the maximum frequency at the start of the waveform (systolic upstroke) indicating plug flow. Late in diastole the Doppler shifted frequencies start to spread out, indicating a change towards parabolic flow (see also Fig. 16.2).

plug flow during systolic acceleration and parabolic flow during diastole. The umbilical artery normally demonstrates parabolic flow throughout the cardiac cycle. Plug flow can be recognised in the Doppler spectrum by all the frequencies being clustered close to the maximum frequency waveform (Fig. 16.3) whilst parabolic flow shows frequencies evenly distributed from the level of the vessel wall filter to the maximum frequency, thus filling the waveform (Fig. 16.4).

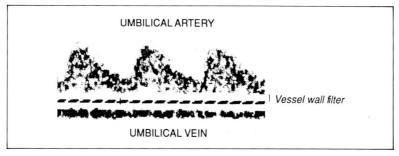

Fig. 16.4 Doppler sonogram from the umbilical artery and vein. The Doppler shifted frequencies recorded from the vein are evenly distributed indicating parabolic flow. The area above the baseline that is free of signal is due to the vessel wall filter removing the low frequency signals caused by movement of the vessel wall.

Ideally the spectrum should consist of Doppler frequencies produced only by axial blood velocity in the vessel of interest. However, the spectrum is always contaminated by other components. Many of these components are unavoidable, such as divergences of the ultrasound beam as it travels through different tissues, or slight spectral distortion due to differences amongst the velocity directions of dispersing erythrocytes. These components of contamination, however, are minor, and a more important source of contamination is caused by Doppler shifts attributable to the pulsatile movements of the vessel walls.

The vessel wall filter

Doppler shifts due to vessel walls are low in frequency but high in intensity. They have an amplitude which is many times higher than the echoes from the erythrocytes because the acoustic mismatch between the vessel wall and blood is much greater than that between the red cell–plasma interface. In order to remove these low frequency Doppler signals generated by the vessel walls, a high pass filter (or wall thump filter) may be used. Initial studies on fetal vessels used a filter of 600 Hz with a 2 MHz Doppler frequency but it has subsequently been shown that this removed low frequency Doppler shifted signals generated by red blood cells and led to a serious miscalculation of average Doppler shift. Filters of 50–200 Hz are now generally used. The most important error caused by high pass filters is to eliminate low velocities occurring at the end of diastole. Nevertheless, manufacturers use high pass filters for very good reasons and whenever Doppler frequencies are substantially above 200 Hz there is nothing to be gained by switching the filter to 50 Hz as harmful vessel motion signals might contaminate an otherwise good signal. Therefore, high pass filters should be used at their highest value and only switched to 50 Hz when necessary.

DOPPLER FLOWMETERS

These are instruments for acquiring, displaying and analysing Doppler waveforms.

The continuous wave flowmeter

The most simple Doppler device is the continuous wave flowmeter, the basic elements of which are illustrated in Figure 16.5.

The master oscillator produces a sinusoidal waveform which is amplified and is used to drive the transmitting transducer at its resonating frequency. The consequent ultrasonic beam hits the moving targets (erythrocytes) which produce reflected and back scattered

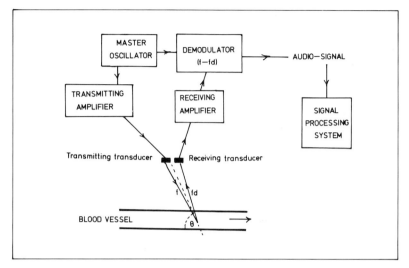

Fig. 16.5 Diagram illustrating the basic components of a continuous wave Doppler system. Essentially, the master oscillator, transmitting amplifier and transducer produce the signal. The returning signal is received by a separate transducer, amplified and passed to the demodulator. This is then compared to the original signal and the difference is displayed as the Doppler shifted waveform.

echoes, some of which will eventually return to the receiving transducer. These are amplified and presented to the Doppler demodulator which compares the frequency of the received signals with a replica of the transmitted signal. The output from the demodulator is the Doppler difference waveform.

For a continuous wave flowmeter a particle moving with a constant velocity across the beam produces a Doppler frequency spread that is inversely proportional to the beam width; that is, the narrower the beam width the wider the spectrum. However, even a single particle travelling at a constant velocity through the beam of a continuous wave flowmeter produces a complete spectrum of Doppler shifted frequencies. This spectral broadening limits the velocity resolution of the Doppler device. Simple continuous wave flowmeters are not limited by the maximum velocity that can be measured and, as they do not usually use real-time imaging, they are relatively cheap (approximately 15–20% of the price of duplex, pulsed Doppler systems). Their major disadvantage, however, is their inability to discriminate in range. The continuous wave transmission creates an ultrasonic beam which occupies the complete diffraction pattern of the transducer. Any target moving within this beam will contribute to the final Doppler output. In clinical use it is sometimes impossible to separate signals from vessels at different depths.

Pulsed Doppler flowmeters

Pulsed Doppler combines the range discriminating capabilities of a pulsed echo system with the velocity detection properties of a Doppler system.

The sample volume

The sample volume can best be visualised as a region at some distance in front of the transducer from which all returning echoes must have originated. The dimensions of the sample volume are defined axially by the pulse length and laterally by the beam width of the ultrasonic beam (see 'Lateral resolution', Ch. 15). If ultrasound travels at a constant velocity, then following transmission the sample volume effectively moves away from the transducer face at half that velocity since the pulse has to travel both to and from the target. By choosing to sample only those Doppler components which return after a preset, constant delay from transmission it is possible to interrogate only those targets moving at a particular range from the transducer. The pulsed Doppler ultrasound interrogates the target only once every pulse repetition period and this defines the rate at which data is collected and thus the maximum frequency at which the Doppler waveform can be updated.

The components of a pulsed Doppler system

Figure 16.6 shows the basic elements of the pulsed Doppler system. In this case, although the master oscillator still generates a sinusoidal waveform at the resonating frequency of the transducer, the transmission gate only allows passage of a few cycles once every pulsed repetition period. The delay gate generates a time delay which is used to sample echoes from a selected depth. Returning echoes are then sampled by opening the range gate and feeding the echoes into a demodulator which compares the received frequency with the transmitted frequency. Each gated return echo produces an output from the demodulator which is stored until the next echo is received. This so-called 'sample and hold' technique produces a smooth output waveform which must be filtered to eliminate the sampling or pulse repetition frequency.

Velocity limitations

The upper limit of frequency shift which can be detected by the pulsed Doppler flowmeter is limited by the sampling process. The Doppler waveform has to be reconstructed from a series of samples taken at regular intervals and the maximum Doppler frequency that can be detected is one-half of the pulsed repetition frequency (Nyquist theory). If higher frequency signals are present then the sampled

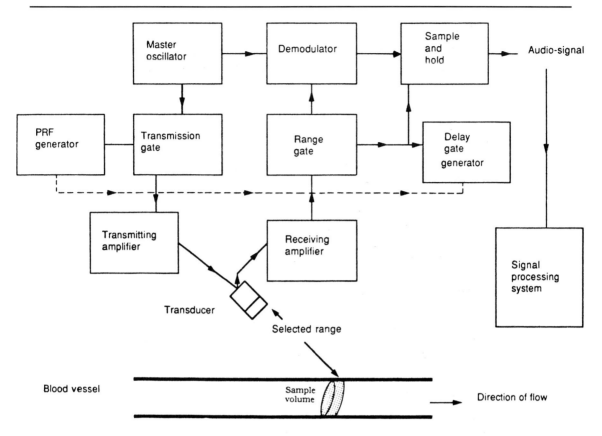

Fig. 16.6 The components of a pulsed Doppler system (see text for explanation).

waveform cannot be reconstructed correctly and a phenomenon known as aliasing occurs (see Figs 16.7 & 16.8). This is the same effect that causes wagon wheels to appear to rotate backwards on the cinema or television screen.

Range-velocity limitations

In addition to maximum velocity limitations, pulsed Doppler systems are also subject to maximum range limitations. The range restrictions occur because it is necessary to wait for the returning echo to have been received from the most distant target before a further pulse of ultrasound is transmitted. This affects the maximum velocity because the deeper the target the lower the pulse repetition frequency (PRF) and the lower the maximum detectable blood velocity. Major fetal vessels are generally located within 15 cm of the surface of the maternal abdomen and the peak systolic velocities recorded from the descending

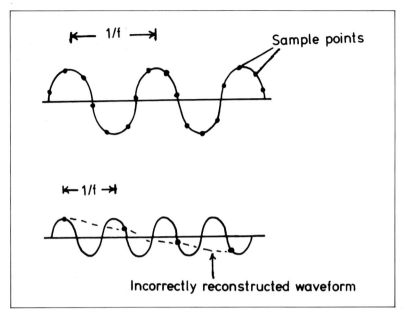

Fig. 16.7 Illustration of the aliasing artifact. In the upper diagram the waveform is sampled sufficiently frequently to allow a correct reconstruction of the waveform. In the lower diagram the infrequent sampling leads to an incorrect reconstruction (dotted line). The results of this are illustrated in Figure 16.8.

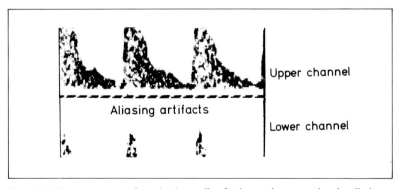

Fig. 16.8 The screen output from the descending fetal aorta demonstrating the aliasing artifact.

aorta can approach 1.5 m/s so that with angles of insonation from 45–55° the optimum PRF is 5–7.5 kHz with ultrasound frequencies of 2–3 MHz. For pulse repetition frequencies of up to 2.5 kHz it is possible to interlace Doppler and real-time ultrasound such that a simultaneous real-time image may be displayed (duplex, pulsed Doppler ultrasound). At pulsed repetition frequencies higher than

2.5 kHz the real-time screen has to be frozen to record the Doppler signals. Most systems have a means of updating the real-time picture about once every second, although sophisticated computerised scanners can present real-time images and Doppler signals simultaneously. For optimum Doppler signals, however, the real-time image must always be frozen.

Table 16.1 indicates the relative importance of various criteria in choosing continuous wave and pulsed Doppler equipment.

Table 16.1 Choosing Doppler equipment

Criteria	Relative importance (0–5)
Continuous wave equipment	
1. 4 MHz continuous wave pencil probe	5
2. Real-time spectral analyser	5
3. Large spectral memory	4
4. Automatic index calculation	3
5. Ability to verify accuracy of maximum frequency outline	4
6. Hand calculation facility	2*
7. Colour spectrum	3
8. Sensitive Doppler with clear, undistorted audible signal	5
9. High pass filter adjustable down to 50 Hz	5
10. Power output of less than 100 mW/cm^2	4
Pulsed Doppler equipment	
Additional features to the continuous wave equipment are:	
1. Offset Doppler for vessels	5
2. Co-axial Doppler for heart and cerebral vessels	5
3. Pulsed Doppler transducer 2–3 MHz	5
4. Depth of 3–12 cm	5
5. Switchable from continuous wave to pulsed wave	3
6. Duplex system	3
7. Pulsed wave with power output of less than 100 mW/cm^2	5
8. Ease of adjustment of sample volume	3
9. Automatic calculation of velocity from vessel diameter and angle	3
10. Automated volume flow calculations	2

* May be more important if automatic maximum frequency is not superimposed upon a spectral analysis display.

PROCESSING DOPPLER SHIFTED SIGNALS

Introduction

Waveforms (for example, electrocardiographic signals) are normally displayed by plotting the amplitude vertically and time horizontally. Doppler signals, however, are displayed by plotting the Doppler frequency vertically (Fig. 16.9). A single Doppler shifted waveform may be displayed, but more usually a complete spectrum of frequencies is shown against time.

The power spectrum

Figure 16.10 illustrates how Doppler insonation of a blood vessel produces a frequency spectrum. The Doppler power spectrum derived from the Doppler signal back-scattered by flowing blood is shown in the lower part of the diagram and because a velocity profile exists across the vessel diameter the Doppler spectrum exists from low frequencies corresponding to echoes from slow moving cells near the vessel walls, to high frequency components generated by blood moving at high velocity along the axis of the vessel. The power spectral density (grey scale of a single spectral line) is an indicator of the volume of blood flowing at a given velocity. It can be further shown that mean blood velocity is directly related by the Doppler equation to the mean frequency which can be computed from the power spectrum. Attempts at determining velocity (or volume flow) must therefore start with a demonstration of an adequate Doppler power spectrum.

The Doppler frequency spectrum

In order to give some idea of the required capabilities of Doppler flowmeters it is useful to examine the properties of the Doppler shift spectrum. Using a 2.5 MHz ultrasound probe to insonate the fetal aorta with an angle of about 40°, the Doppler spectrum would be expected to extend up to a frequency of about 6 kHz corresponding to a peak

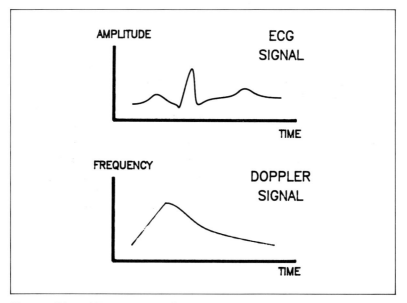

Fig. 16.9 Diagram illustrating the different presentation of a Doppler waveform (*frequency* against time) compared to the ECG signal.

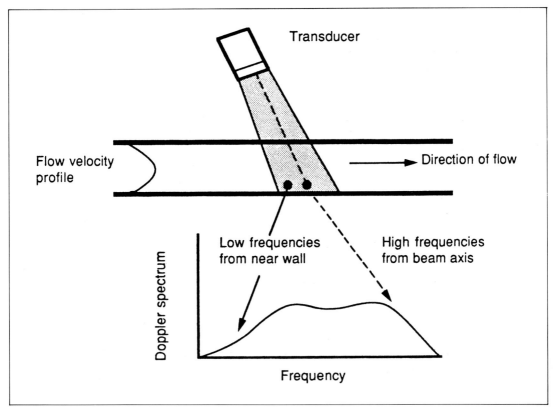

Fig. 16.10 Illustration of how the Doppler shifted frequency power spectrum is obtained.

velocity of about 1.6 m/s during the maximum systolic phase. Furthermore, the blood would accelerate from almost complete rest at the end of diastole up to this peak velocity in a time interval of less than 0.1 s. The Doppler signal frequency analyser must therefore be able to accommodate frequencies up to 10 kHz and must be capable of updating the analysis at a rate of at least 100 spectra per second. However, if lower ultrasonic frequencies are used to investigate more slowly moving venous blood it would be better to use lower range analysis frequencies placed closer together to maintain the required frequency (and therefore velocity resolution). Thus a switchable frequency analyser would be more useful where multiple purpose instrumentation is needed.

Real-time spectrum analysis

A real-time spectrum analyser is an instrument which measures the power of all the frequencies contained in the Doppler signal.

Furthermore it separates forward (that is blood flowing towards the transducer) and reverse signals into separate channels. The simple method of performing spectrum analysis is real-time compression. The Doppler signal is digitised and scanned rapidly (200 times per second) by a sweeping filter which measures the power of each individual frequency. The method most commonly employed is known as Fast Fourier Transform (FFT). The principles and mathematics are beyond the scope of this chapter but the method essentially is the same as time compression in that the signal is digitised and analysed by rapid scanning. The characteristics of an analyser which are important to the user are the speed of operation and the number of separate frequencies which can be resolved. For obstetric use a sampling time of 5 ms (200 per second) is desirable with a frequency resolution of at least 64 bins per channel, although most analysers offer at least 128 frequency bins.

Real-time spectral analysis is essential in obstetrics use, as the Doppler signals are often complex and contain frequencies emanating from more than one vessel. Providing the user can see the spectrum displayed in real time, these artifacts can be detected. More importantly, as most analysers now perform automatic calculations, the user must be able to judge whether the signal selected by the analyser is valid or whether the reading should be discarded because of artifact.

Automatic calculations performed by the analyser are performed mostly on the maximum frequency outline. In order to recognise this the analyser inspects each of the frequency bins in turn and determines the highest frequency at which there is a signal. This simple approach only works on near perfect waveforms with a high signal to noise ratio, so in practice the analyser's microprocessor imposes several conditions which must be satisfied before it validates the maximum frequency. The maximum frequency is usually superimposed upon the spectral display so that the user can judge whether it is a true representation. Early analysers were incapable of performing this task and the operator was required to draw round the maximum frequency outline using a computer graphics pencil, or a light pen. These manual methods could only be performed upon stored data whereas automatic calculations are performed in real time.

Calculations performed using the maximum frequency outline

When the vascular system is subject to pulses from the heart its behaviour is very similar to mechanical springs subject to a weight and some kind of damper. Everyday examples such as car suspension springs or guitar strings perform some kind of damped oscillation in response to being disturbed, and blood velocity waveforms exhibit similar characteristics. The spring is represented in blood vessels by their compliance, and dampening by factors such as blood viscosity, vessel length and luminal diameter. Thus a typical blood velocity waveform will have a maximum at the peak of systole followed by diastolic frequencies which might, in one extreme, oscillate to the reverse flow direction before falling to zero, or in the other extreme may fall gently until the next systole. There are several indices which attempt to describe these variations in the waveforms and the most commonly used are illustrated in Figure 13.3. All these indices are independent of the angle between the Doppler beam and the vessel.

The pulsatility index (PI) was originally described as the difference between the most positive (or highest value) and the most negative (or lowest value) over one cardiac cycle, divided by the mean value. In bi-directional waveforms the most negative value is found in the reverse channel. The mean (or time average mean, TAM) is the mean frequency averaged over one cardiac cycle. The concept of this index is that the more pulsatile the waveform, the greater the difference between the positive and negative peaks and the higher the value of the PI. Flow velocity waveforms from the uteroplacental circulation are rarely (if ever) bi-directional and reverse flow in the umbilical artery only occurs when the fetus is in extremis, so simple indices have been more widely applied to such waveforms.

The A:B (or S:D) ratio is simple and describes the rate at which flow velocities fall away during diastole. This closely corresponds to the peripheral resistance to blood flow beyond the measurement point. The resistance index (RI) makes use of the same two points as the A:B ratio but expresses the values in a more convenient form.

Peripheral resistance cannot be directly measured by means of Doppler waveforms but increasing peripheral resistance causes a diminution and then a loss of frequencies in end-diastole. In vessels that supply vascular beds of muscles, increasing peripheral resistance causes an increase in pulsatility and consequently a rise in the PI. In obstetric practice reverse flow rarely occurs and as peripheral resistance is further increased the systolic peak decreases in amplitude thus giving a decrease in the PI. If the values of the PI are considered in isolation, this worsening situation can result in a false sense of security. Furthermore, calculation of the PI requires a complete and accurate maximum frequency waveform in order to calculate the time-averaged mean frequency.

As end-diastolic frequencies disappear, point B becomes zero, so the A:B ratio becomes infinity whilst the RI becomes unity. In all situations where end-diastolic frequencies are lost it is best to describe this in words rather than using indices.

Frequency, velocity and volume calculations

The maximum frequency waveform is relatively simple to derive from the Doppler spectrum and describes the variation in the fastest moving red blood cells, which occupy the centre of the vessel. In order to calculate blood flow an estimate of the mean of all the velocities recorded throughout the cardiac cycle is needed. This parameter is known as the Intensity Weighted Mean Frequency (IWMF). The IWMF is the sum of the product of the square of the amplitude of each frequency (a) and that frequency (f), divided by the sum of the square of the amplitudes:

$$IWMF = \Sigma_0^{max} a^2 . f / \Sigma_0^{max} a^2$$

The amplitude of the signal must be squared when making this calculation because the power or intensity of each frequency is proportional to the square of the signal amplitude or voltage. Contamination by signals from other vessels invalidates IWMF because the mean of all signals is calculated, whereas the maximum frequency waveform is much more reliable in this respect.

Velocity calculations

If the angle between the Doppler beam and the blood vessel is known then the frequency can be converted into actual blood velocity (see 'Doppler principle'). Velocity measurements have not achieved popularity in obstetric use because of the errors of accurately measuring the angle of insonation. In obstetric practice velocity measurements can only be reliably obtained from the descending fetal aorta.

Volume flow calculations

In order to calculate volume flow accurately, estimation of the IWMF, the angle of insonation and the vessel diameter are required. Measurement of vessel diameter is difficult because:

1. Diameter measurements are usually made by means of on-screen calipers to the nearest millimetre.
2. The diameter has to be squared in order to derive the cross-sectional area of the vessel, hence any error in measurement will be squared.
3. The cross-section of the vessel is not necessarily round, for example the descending fetal aorta tends to be flattened in an anteroposterior direction.
4. The cross-sectional diameter of the vessel may change between systole and diastole.

Overall, errors in the vessel diameter measurements, measurements of angle, and calculation of IWMF lead to errors of up to 30% in volume flow calculation in the obstetric field.

Duplex, pulsed Doppler ultrasound

These systems utilise a real-time transducer (commonly 3.5 MHz linear array) together with a Doppler transducer (either 2.0 or 4.0 MHz). Scanner timing circuits provide one scanning period for each line and an additional period to display an electronic caliper. To display the Doppler vector on the two-dimensional image obtained from the real-time scanner a further period of 1 ms needs to be generated and a switch multiplexer has to be inserted between the scanner and the oscilloscope. Since the pulsed Doppler and pulsed linear array interfere with one another if operated at the same time, one can only have either the scanner or the pulsed Doppler. The operating sequence is therefore modified so that the memory control sequence has an intermediate position between real time and frame freeze. In this position (called auto-update) the frozen picture is electronically refreshed once every second and the pulsed Doppler momentarily switched off. This enables continuous monitoring of the registration between the Doppler sample and the vessel position. This sequence is activated by the frame-freeze foot-switch of the real-time scanner, which now has three sequence operations instead of two. At low pulse repetition rates (less than 2.5 kHz) it is possible to interlace the real-time image and the Doppler to allow simultaneous display (for further details see Teague et al 1985 — see Further Reading). Such instruments are needed in order to obtain maximum frequency waveforms or velocity measurements from fetal vessels such as the descending aorta, the fetal cerebral circulation and the fetal renal artery.

COLOUR FLOW DOPPLER ULTRASOUND

Colour flow mapping consists of a colour coded map superimposed upon a real-time B-mode image. In each real-time frame the mean Doppler frequency (or occasionally the variance of the spread of the Doppler frequencies) is calculated and displayed by an appropriate choice of colour. The mean Doppler frequency is usually calculated within a colour flow pixel as a spatial average. Variance is calculated from the distribution of all the Doppler frequencies and indicates the degree of turbulence within a colour flow pixel; the greater the turbulence the greater the variance.

Several colour maps are available on modern machines but a common scheme represents flow towards the transducer as red and flow away as blue. The magnitude of the mean Doppler frequency within a colour flow pixel is usually represented by the strength of the colour (known as the colour saturation).

The great advantage of colour flow mapping is that the signal relies only upon the presence of a Doppler signal so that small blood vessels (for example those in the fetal circle of Willis) may be visualised even though they are below the spatial resolution of the real-time image. Errors in interpretation may occur, however, as each colour flow pixel in a single scanning line is sampled by transmitted pulses. Hence, the Nyquist theory applies and if the mean Doppler frequency is more than half the pulse repetition frequency then aliasing occurs (see 'Pulsed Doppler flowmeters'). The wrapround effect leads to a blue contamination of a red colour map in areas of very high flow towards the probe.

Colour flow mapping is dependent upon the angle of insonation, hence blood moving at the same velocity may appear in different colours in differing parts of a curved vessel. Furthermore, absence of colour does not necessarily indicate absence of flow as no colour will be displayed if the beam is at right angles to the vessel.

APPENDIX ONE
Differential diagnosis of common problems

CAUSES OF SMALL FOR DATES

- Wrong dates
- Missed abortion
- Fetal death
- Intrauterine growth retardation
- Oligohydramnios
- Spontaneous rupture of membranes.

CAUSES OF BLEEDING

First trimester
- Abortion
  — incomplete
  — missed
  — threatened
- Hydatidiform mole
- Ectopic gestation.

Second and third trimesters
- Placenta praevia
- Abruption
- Hydatidiform mole
- Marginal sinus rupture.

CAUSES OF LARGE FOR DATES

- Incorrect dates
- Multiple pregnancy. If the fetuses are of different sizes the pregnancy should be dated by the measurement of the larger fetus
- Fetal macrosomia
- Uterine fibroids
- Ovarian cysts
- Polyhydramnios
- End-stage hydrocephaly.

CAUSES OF LOWER ABDOMINAL PAIN

First and second trimester
- Ectopic gestation
- Large corpus luteal cyst (more than 5 cm)
- Abortion
- Degeneration of a fibroid.

Third trimester
- Abruption
- Preterm labour
- Degeneration of a fibroid.

APPENDIX TWO
Differential diagnosis of abnormal ultrasound findings and commonly associated abnormalities

CAUSES OF POLYHYDRAMNIOS

- Multiple pregnancy
- Fetal abnormality
  — impaired fetal swallowing, e.g. as in some cases of anencephaly
  — bowel atresias, e.g. duodenal atresia
  — impaired absorption of amniotic fluid by fetal bowel, e.g. some cases of omphalocoele
  — some limb reduction deformities
  — cystic adenomatoid malformation
  — hydrops fetalis, from any cause
- Maternal diabetes mellitus
- Maternal uraemia.

CAUSES OF OLIGOHYDRAMNIOS

- Spontaneous rupture of the membranes
- Intrauterine growth retardation
- Lesions of the fetal urinary tract, e.g. renal agenesis, urethral stenosis.

CAUSES OF A MASS WITHIN THE FETUS

Head
- Encephalocoele
- Teratoma.

Neck
- Cystic hygroma
- Thyroid goitre.

Chest
- Diaphragmatic hernia which may contain liver or spleen
- Ectopia cordis, i.e. the heart being outside the chest cavity
- Cystic adenomatoid malformation.

Abdomen
- Infantile polycystic kidneys
- Omphalocoele
- Gastroschisis
- Umbilical hernia
- Teratoma
- Echogenic bowel e.g. from cystic fibrosis.

Spine
- Spina bifida
- Sacrococcygeal teratoma.

АНТ АНТ

CAUSES OF ECHO FREE AREAS WITHIN THE FETUS

Fetal head
- Hydrocephaly
- Hydranencephaly
- Holoprosencephaly
- Porencephalic cyst
- Choroid plexus cyst
- Dandy–Walker syndrome
- Arachnoid cyst.

Chest
- Diaphragmatic hernia
- Lung cyst (congenital cystic adenomatoid malformation)
- Pleural effusion
- Pericardial effusion.

Abdomen
Normal
Stomach, bladder, gallbladder, renal pelvis, umbilical vein, portal vein, aorta and inferior vena cava.

Single
Solitary cyst of the kidney, liver, ovary and mesentery. Unilateral pelvi-ureteric junction obstruction. Enlarged bladder due to urethral atresia or stenosis.

Double
Duodenal atresia
Bilateral pelvi-ureteric junction obstruction
Choledochal cyst.

Triple
Jejunal atresia
Obstructive uropathy, in which case the echo free areas are from the bladder and the hydronephroses.

Multiple
Multicystic or polycystic kidneys
Obstructive uropathy
Bowel obstruction
Ascites.

COMMONLY ASSOCIATED FETAL ABNORMALITIES

Abnormality	Associations
● Achondroplasia	Spina bifida Microcephaly Infantile polycystic kidneys
● Arrhinencephaly	Facial anomalies (cyclops, median cleft lip)
● Cloacal extrophy	Spina bifida Omphalocoele
● Diaphragmatic hernia	Spina bifida Hydronephroses
● Duodenal atresia	Down syndrome (about 30%)
● Gastroschisis	Usually none
● Hydrocephaly	Spina bifida Infantile polycystic kidneys Polydactyly
● Imperforate anus	Cloacal extrophy Trisomy 18 and 21 Urinary tract anomalies
● Obstructive uropathy	Chromosome anomalies (about 20%) Spina bifida Bowel abnormalities
● Omphalocoele	Polyhydramnios Cardiac anomalies (about 30%) Chromosome anomalies (about 30%) Neural tube defects (about 30%)
● Renal dysplasia	Encephalocoele Hydrocephaly Microcephaly Polydactyly (Any of the above with renal dysplasia is known as Meckel's sydrome)

APPENDIX THREE
Markers of chromosomal abnormality

MARKER	KARYOTYPE	PROBABLE RISK
Agenesis of corpus callosum	trisomy 13	5%
Cardiac abnormalities	trisomy 13, 18, 21 triploidy	15%
Choroid plexus cysts	trisomy 18, 21	<1%
Clasped or overlapping fingers	trisomy 18	?
Clinodactyly	trisomy 21 Fanconi's syndrome	?
Cystic hygroma	45 XO trisomy 21, 18, 13	90%
Diaphragmatic hernia	trisomy 18	15%
Dilated ureters	trisomy 18, 21	30%
Duodenal atresia	trisomy 21	30%
Holoprosencephaly	trisomy 13, 18	90%
Hydrocephaly	triploidy	<1%
Lateral facial cleft	trisomy 18	<1%
Median facial cleft	trisomy 21, 13	50%
Microcephaly	some chromosomal deletions	?
Multicystic dysplastic kidneys	trisomy 18	?
Non-immune hydrops	45 XO	?
Non-immune hydrops and cystic hygroma	45 XO	99%
Nuchal fat pad	trisomy 21, 45 XO	?
Obstructive uropathy (low)	trisomy 18, 13	20%
Omphalocoele	trisomy 13, 18	30%
Radial aplasia/thumb hypoplasia	trisomy 13	90%
Rocker bottom feet	trisomy 18	50%
Sandal gap	trisomy 21	?
Single umbilical artery	trisomy 18, 21	5%
Syndactyly/polydactyly	trisomy 13 triploidy	?

Note: The figures are the best estimate that can be obtained from the prenatal diagnosis literature. Those markers with a '?' probably have a low association and on their own do not currently warrant karyotyping. Combinations of markers increase the risk by an unknown amount, but we would offer karyotyping if two or more markers were present, e.g. a nuchal fat pad with a sandal gap.

291

APPENDIX FOUR
Estimation of gestational age from CRL, BPD and FL

The following tables are recommended by the British Medical Ultrasound Society. They should be used to establish gestational age *only* in the following circumstances:

- When the woman's menstrual dates are unknown or unreliable (see p. 77)
- When measurements of the biometric parameters obtained before 24 weeks gestation fall outside the data reference range of the charts given for each parameter.

They should also be used in conjunction with the correct technique of measurement, details of which can be found as follows: crown–rump length (p. 55); biparietal diameter (p. 80); femur length (p. 90).

References (with kind permission)

Table A. Robinson H P, Fleming J E E 1975 A critical evaluation of sonar crown–rump length measurements. British Journal of Obstetrics and Gynaecology 82: 702–710

Table B. Hadlock F P, Deter R L, Harrist R B, Park S K 1982 Fetal biparietal diameter: a critical re-evaluation of the relationship to menstrual age by means of real-time ultrasound. Journal of Ultrasound in Medicine 1: 97–104

Table C. Warda A H, Deter R L, Rossavik I K 1985 Fetal femur length: a critical re-evaluation of the relationship to menstrual age. Obstetrics and Gynecology 66: 69–75

A. Estimation of gestational age from crown–rump length

CRL (mm)	GA	
	Weeks	Days
4	6	0
6	6	3
8	6	6
10	7	1
12	7	4
14	8	0
16	8	2
18	8	4
20	8	5
22	9	0
24	9	2
26	9	3
28	9	5
30	9	6
32	10	1
34	10	2
36	10	3
38	10	5
40	11	0
42	11	1
44	11	2
46	11	3
48	11	4
50	11	5
52	11	6
54	12	1
56	12	2
58	12	3
60	12	4
62	12	5
64	12	6
66	13	0
68	13	1
70	13	2
72	13	3
74	13	4
76	13	5
78	13	6
80	14	0

B. Estimation of gestational age from biparietal diameter

BPD (mm)	GA	
	Weeks	Days
20	12	2
22	12	5
24	13	2
26	13	6
28	14	3
30	15	0
32	15	4
34	16	1
36	16	6
38	17	3
40	18	0
42	18	4
44	19	2
46	19	6
48	20	4
50	21	1
52	21	6
54	22	4
56	23	1
58	23	6
60	24	4
62	25	2
64	26	0
66	26	6
68	27	4
70	28	2
72	29	1
74	30	0
76	30	5
78	31	4
80	32	3
82	33	2
84	34	2
86	35	1
88	36	0
90	37	0
92	38	0
94	39	0
96	40	0
98	41	0
100	42	0

C. Estimation of gestational age from femur length

FL (mm)	GA	
	Weeks	Days
10	13	1
12	13	5
14	14	2
16	15	0
18	15	4
20	16	1
22	16	6
24	17	4
26	18	2
28	19	0
30	19	5
32	20	3
34	21	1
36	21	6
38	22	5
40	23	3
42	24	2
44	25	1
46	25	6
48	26	5
50	27	4
52	28	3
54	29	2
56	30	1
58	31	0
60	31	6
62	32	6
64	33	5
66	34	4
68	35	3
70	36	3
72	37	2
74	38	1
76	39	0
78	39	6
80	40	6

APPENDIX FIVE

Full Size Charts

The charts in this section include these recommended by BMUS (see Further reading) and are full size for ease of use within the department.

References (with kind permission)

Chart A. Hadlock F P, Deter R L, Harrist R B, Park S K 1982 Fetal biparietal diameter: a critical re-evaluation of the relationship to menstrual age by means of real-time ultrasound. Journal of Ultrasound in Medicine 1: 97–104
Chart B. Hadlock F P, Deter R L, Harrist R B, Park S K 1982 Fetal head circumference: relation to menstrual age. American journal of Radiology 38: 647–653
Chart C. Deter R L, Harrist R B, Hadlock F P, Carpenter R J 1982 Fetal head and abdominal circumferences: II. A critical re-evaluation of the relationship to menstrual age. Journal of Clinical Ultrasound 10: 365–372
Chart D. Warda A H, Deter R L, Rossavik I K 1985 Fetal femur length: a critical re-evaluation of the relationship to menstrual age. Obstetrics and Gynecology 66: 69–75
Charts E, F and G. Romero R, Pilu G, Jeanty P, Ghidini A, Hobbins J 1988 Prenatal diagnosis of congenital anomalies. Appleton and Lange, Charts E & F: p. 323, Chart G: p. 324
Chart H. Modified from: Campbell S, Thoms A, 1977 British Journal of Obstetrics and Gynaecology 84: 165–174.
Chart I. Pearce J M 1992 Doppler ultrasound in perinatal medicine. Oxford University Press, Oxford.

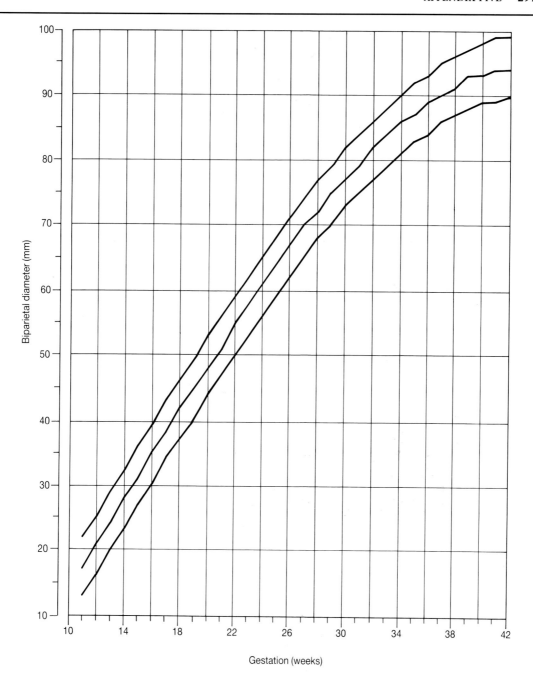

Chart A Growth of biparietal diameter.

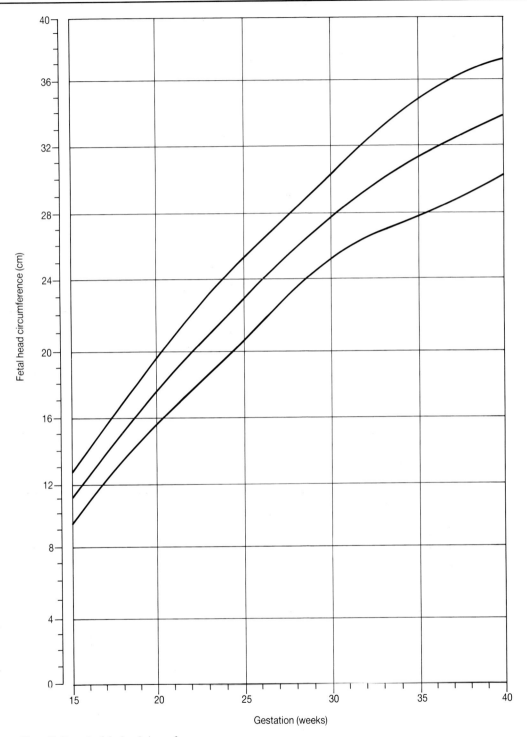

Chart B Growth of the head circumference.

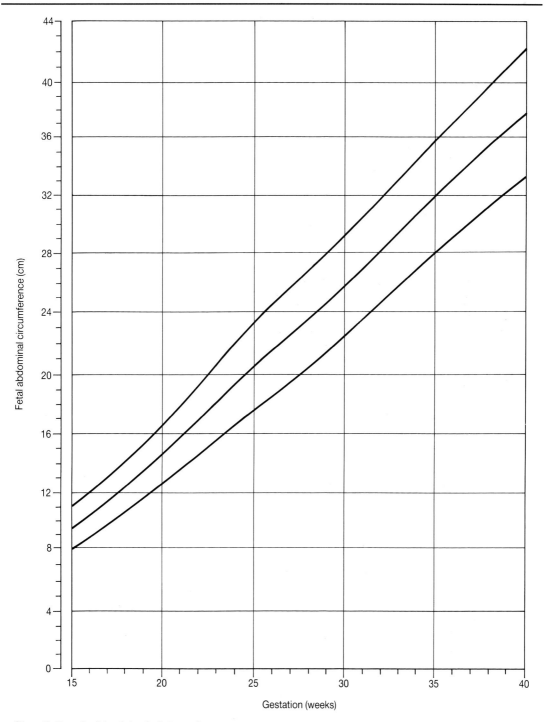

Chart C Growth of the abdominal circumference.

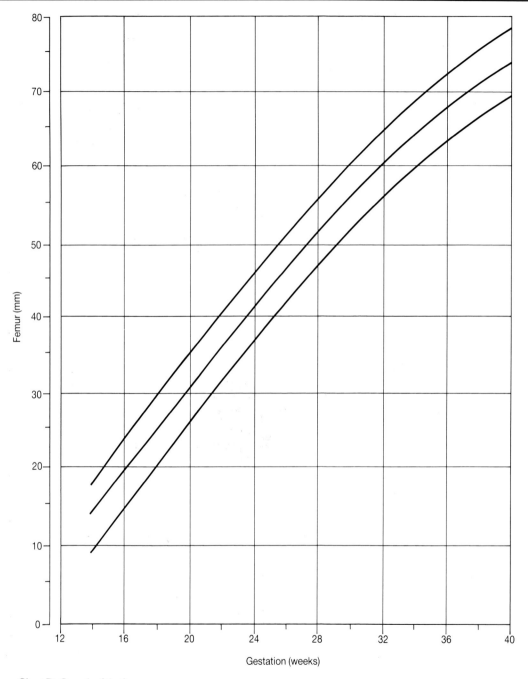

Chart D Growth of the femur.

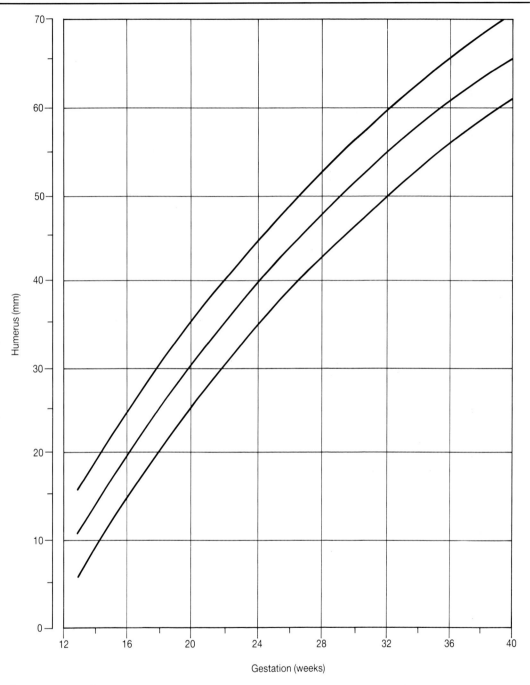

Chart E Growth of the humerus.

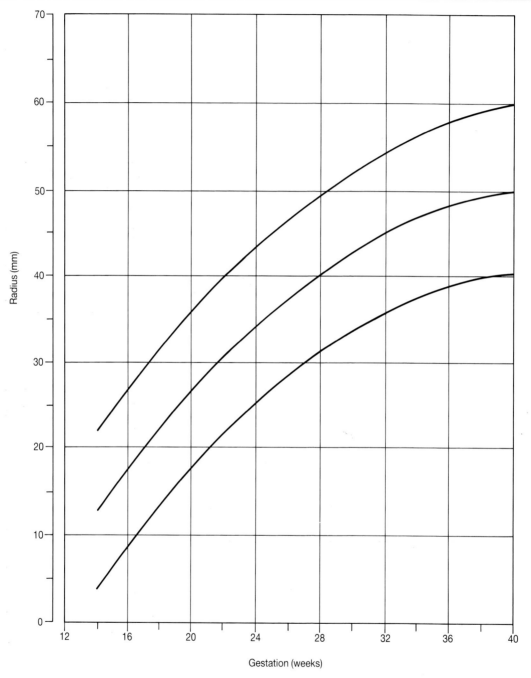

Chart F Growth of the radius.

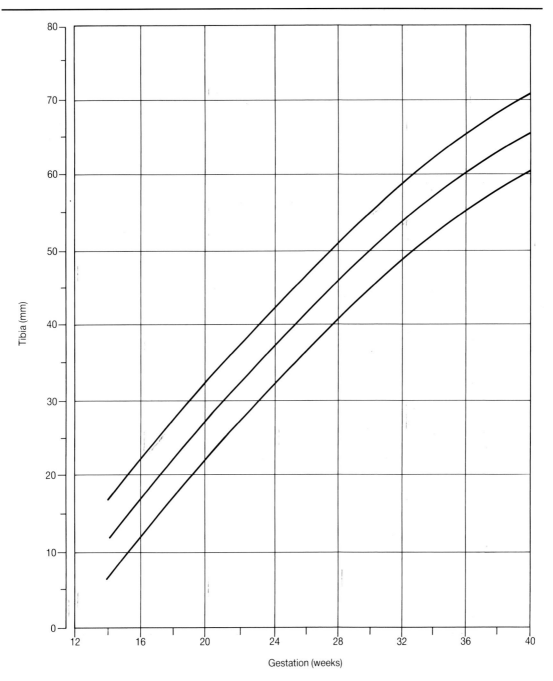

Chart G Growth of the tibia.

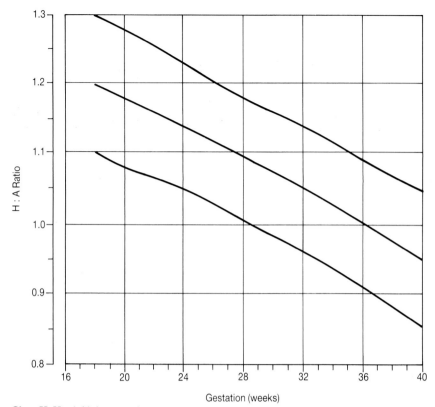

Chart H Head:Abdomen ratio.

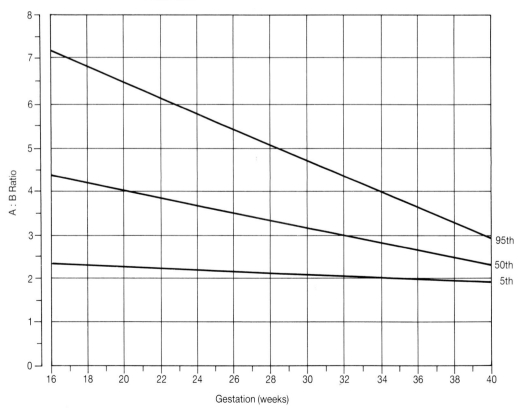

Chart I The umbilical artery A:B ratio.

APPENDIX SIX
Estimation of fetal weight from BPD, AC and FL

A. Estimation of fetal weight from measurements of the BPD and abdominal circumference. (Adapted from Shepard M J, Richards V A and Berkowitz R L (1982) American Journal of Obstetrics and Gynecology; by Jeanty P and Romero R in Obstetrical Ultrasound, by kind permission of McGraw-Hill.)

Abdominal Circumference (mm)

BPD (mm)	40	45	50	55	60	65	70	75	80	85	90	95	100	105	110	115	120	125	130	135	140	145	150
30	80	83	87	91	95	99	104	108	113	118	123	129	135	141	147	154	161						
31	83	86	90	94	98	103	107	112	117	122	128	133	139	145	152	159	166	173	181				
32			93	97	102	106	111	116	121	126	132	138	144	150	157	164	171	178	186				
33			97	101	105	110	115	120	125	130	136	142	148	155	162	169	176	184	192				
34			100	104	109	114	119	124	129	135	141	147	153	160	167	174	182	190	198	206	215		
35					113	118	123	128	134	139	145	152	158	165	172	180	187	195	204	213	222		
36					117	122	127	132	138	144	150	157	163	170	178	185	193	202	210	219	229		
37					121	126	131	137	143	149	155	162	169	176	183	191	199	208	217	226	235	245	256
38							136	142	148	154	160	167	174	182	189	197	206	214	223	233	243	253	263
39							141	146	153	159	166	173	180	187	195	203	212	221	230	240	250	260	271

BPD (mm)	70	75	80	85	90	95	100	105	110	115	120	125	130	135	140	145	150	155	160	165	170	175	180
40	145	152	158	164	171	178	186	193	202	210	219	228	237	247	257	268	279						
41			163	170	177	184	192	200	208	217	226	235	245	255	265	276	288	299	312				
42			169	176	183	190	198	206	215	223	233	242	252	262	273	284	296	308	321				
43			174	182	189	197	205	213	222	231	240	250	260	270	281	293	305	317	330				
44			180	188	195	203	211	220	229	238	247	257	268	279	290	302	314	326	340	353	368		
45					202	210	218	227	236	245	255	265	276	287	299	311	323	336	349	363	378		
46					208	217	225	234	244	253	263	274	285	296	308	320	333	346	359	374	389		
47					215	224	233	242	251	261	271	282	293	305	317	329	342	356	370	384	400	415	432
48							240	250	259	269	280	291	302	314	326	339	352	366	381	395	411	427	444
49							248	258	268	278	289	300	312	324	336	349	363	377	392	407	422	439	456

BPD (mm)	100	105	110	115	120	125	130	135	140	145	150	155	160	165	170	175	180	185	190	195	200	205	210	215	220
50	256	266	276	287	298	309	321	334	346	360	374	388	403	418	434	451	468	486	505						
51			285	296	307	319	331	344	357	370	385	399	414	430	447	464	481	500	519						
52			294	305	317	329	341	354	368	381	396	411	426	443	459	477	495	513	533						
53			304	315	327	339	352	365	379	393	408	423	439	455	472	490	508	527	547	568	589				
54					337	350	363	376	390	405	420	435	451	468	486	504	522	542	562	583	605				
55					348	360	374	388	402	417	432	448	464	482	499	518	537	557	577	598	620				
56					359	372	385	399	414	429	445	461	478	495	513	532	552	572	593	614	637	660	684		
57							397	412	426	442	458	474	492	509	528	547	567	587	609	631	654	677	702		
58							409	424	439	455	471	488	506	524	543	562	583	604	625	648	671	695	720		
59									453	469	485	503	520	539	558	578	599	620	642	665	689	713	739	765	792

BPD (mm) × Abdominal Circumference (mm) — estimated fetal weight

BPD 60–69 (Abdominal Circumference 140–250 mm)

BPD	140	145	150	155	160	165	170	175	180	185	190	195	200	205	210	215	220	225	230	235	240	245	250
60	466	483	500	517	536	554	574	594	615	637	659	683	707	732	758	784	812						
61	480	497	514	532	551	570	590	611	632	654	677	701	725	751	777	804	832						
62			530	548	567	587	607	628	650	672	696	720	745	770	797	825	853	883	913				
63			545	564	583	603	624	645	668	691	714	739	764	790	818	846	875	905	936				
64			561	580	600	621	642	664	686	709	734	759	784	811	839	867	897	927	959				
65					617	638	660	682	705	729	753	779	805	832	860	889	919	950	982	1015	1050		
66					635	657	678	701	725	749	774	800	826	854	882	912	942	974	1006	1040	1075		
67					654	675	698	721	745	769	795	821	848	876	905	935	966	998	1031	1065	1100	1137	1174
68							717	741	765	790	816	843	870	899	928	959	990	1023	1056	1091	1127	1164	1202
69							738	762	786	812	838	865	893	922	952	983	1015	1048	1082	1117	1154	1191	1230

BPD 70–79 (Abdominal Circumference 170–290 mm)

BPD	170	175	180	185	190	195	200	205	210	215	220	225	230	235	240	245	250	255	260	265	270	275	280	285	290
70	758	783	808	834	861	888	917	946	977	1008	1041	1074	1109	1144	1181	1219	1258	1299	1340						
71			830	857	884	912	941	971	1002	1034	1067	1101	1136	1172	1209	1248	1287	1328	1371						
72			853	880	908	936	966	996	1028	1060	1094	1128	1164	1200	1238	1277	1317	1359	1402						
73					932	961	991	1022	1054	1087	1121	1156	1192	1229	1268	1307	1348	1390	1433	1478	1524				
74					958	987	1018	1049	1081	1115	1149	1185	1221	1259	1298	1338	1379	1422	1466	1511	1558				
75					983	1013	1044	1076	1109	1143	1178	1214	1251	1290	1329	1370	1411	1455	1499	1545	1592	1641	1691		
76							1072	1104	1138	1172	1208	1244	1282	1321	1361	1402	1444	1488	1533	1579	1627	1676	1727		
77							1100	1133	1167	1202	1238	1275	1313	1353	1393	1435	1478	1522	1568	1615	1663	1713	1764		
78							1129	1163	1197	1233	1269	1307	1346	1385	1426	1469	1512	1557	1603	1651	1700	1750	1802	1855	1910
79								1228	1264	1301	1339	1379	1419	1461	1503	1547	1593	1639	1688	1737	1788	1840	1894	1950	

BPD 80–89 (Abdominal Circumference 210–330 mm)

BPD	210	215	220	225	230	235	240	245	250	255	260	265	270	275	280	285	290	295	300	305	310	315	320	325	330
80	1260	1296	1334	1373	1412	1453	1495	1539	1583	1629	1677	1725	1775	1827	1880	1934	1990								
81			1367	1407	1447	1488	1531	1575	1620	1667	1715	1764	1814	1866	1920	1975	2032	2090	2150						
82			1402	1441	1482	1524	1568	1612	1658	1705	1753	1803	1854	1907	1961	2017	2074	2133	2193						
83			1437	1477	1519	1561	1605	1650	1697	1744	1793	1843	1895	1948	2003	2059	2117	2176	2237	2300	2365				
84					1556	1599	1643	1689	1736	1784	1834	1885	1937	1991	2046	2103	2161	2221	2282	2346	2411				
85					1594	1638	1683	1729	1776	1825	1875	1927	1979	2034	2090	2147	2206	2266	2328	2392	2458				
86							1723	1770	1818	1867	1918	1970	2023	2078	2134	2192	2252	2313	2375	2440	2506	2574	2644		
87							1764	1811	1860	1910	1961	2014	2068	2123	2180	2238	2298	2360	2423	2488	2555	2623	2694		
88							1806	1854	1903	1954	2005	2059	2113	2169	2227	2286	2346	2408	2472	2538	2605	2674	2745	2817	2892
89									1947	1998	2051	2104	2160	2216	2274	2334	2395	2457	2522	2588	2656	2725	2797	2870	2945

BPD 90–100 (Abdominal Circumference 255–375 mm)

BPD	255	260	265	270	275	280	285	290	295	300	305	310	315	320	325	330	335	340	345	350	355	360	365	370	375
90	2044	2097	2151	2207	2264	2323	2383	2445	2508	2573	2639	2707	2778	2849	2923	2999									
91		2145	2199	2256	2313	2372	2433	2495	2559	2624	2692	2760	2831	2903	2977	3054	3132	3212							
92		2193	2249	2305	2364	2423	2484	2547	2611	2677	2745	2814	2885	2958	3033	3109	3188	3268							
93		2243	2299	2356	2415	2475	2537	2600	2665	2731	2799	2869	2941	3014	3089	3166	3245	3326	3409	3494					
94				2408	2467	2528	2590	2654	2719	2786	2855	2925	2997	3071	3147	3224	3304	3385	3468	3554					
95				2461	2521	2582	2645	2709	2775	2842	2912	2982	3055	3129	3205	3283	3363	3445	3528	3614					
96						2637	2701	2765	2832	2900	2969	3041	3114	3188	3265	3343	3423	3505	3590	3676	3764	3854			
97						2694	2757	2823	2890	2958	3028	3100	3173	3248	3325	3404	3485	3567	3652	3738	3827	3918			
98								2881	2949	3018	3088	3160	3234	3310	3387	3466	3547	3630	3715	3802	3891	3982	4075	4170	
99								2941	3009	3078	3149	3222	3296	3372	3450	3530	3611	3695	3780	3867	3956	4047	4141	4236	
100								3002	3071	3141	3212	3285	3360	3436	3514	3594	3676	3760	3845	3933	4022	4114	4207	4303	4401

N.B. All weights expressed in grams.

B. Estimation of fetal weight from measurements of the femur length and abdominal circumference. (From Hadlock et al (1984) Radiology 150: 535)

FL (mm)	Abdominal Circumference (mm)																				
	200	205	210	215	220	225	230	235	240	245	250	255	260	265	270	275	280	285	290	295	300
40	663	691	720	751	783	816	851	887	925	964	1006	1048	1093	1139	1188	1239	1291	1346	1403	1463	1525
41	680	709	738	769	802	836	871	907	946	986	1027	1070	1115	1162	1211	1262	1315	1371	1429	1489	1551
42	697	726	757	788	821	855	891	928	967	1007	1049	1093	1138	1186	1235	1287	1340	1396	1454	1515	1578
43	715	745	776	808	841	875	912	949	988	1029	1071	1116	1162	1209	1259	1311	1365	1422	1480	1541	1605
44	734	764	795	827	861	896	933	971	1010	1051	1094	1139	1185	1234	1284	1336	1391	1448	1507	1568	1632
45	753	783	815	847	882	917	954	993	1033	1074	1118	1163	1210	1259	1309	1362	1417	1474	1534	1596	1660
46	772	803	835	868	903	939	976	1015	1056	1098	1142	1187	1235	1284	1335	1388	1444	1501	1561	1623	1688
47	792	823	856	889	924	961	999	1038	1079	1122	1166	1212	1260	1310	1361	1415	1471	1529	1589	1652	1717
48	812	844	877	911	947	984	1022	1062	1103	1146	1191	1237	1286	1336	1388	1442	1498	1557	1618	1681	1746
49	833	865	899	933	969	1007	1046	1086	1128	1171	1216	1263	1312	1363	1415	1470	1527	1585	1647	1710	1776
50	855	887	921	956	993	1031	1070	1111	1153	1197	1243	1290	1339	1390	1443	1498	1555	1615	1676	1740	1806
51	877	910	944	980	1016	1055	1095	1136	1179	1223	1269	1317	1367	1418	1471	1527	1584	1644	1706	1770	1837
52	899	933	967	1004	1041	1080	1120	1162	1205	1250	1296	1344	1395	1447	1500	1556	1614	1674	1737	1801	1868
53	922	956	992	1028	1066	1105	1146	1188	1232	1277	1324	1373	1423	1476	1530	1586	1645	1705	1768	1833	1900
54	946	981	1016	1053	1091	1131	1172	1215	1259	1305	1352	1401	1452	1505	1560	1617	1675	1736	1799	1865	1933
55	971	1005	1041	1079	1118	1158	1199	1242	1287	1333	1381	1431	1482	1535	1591	1648	1707	1768	1832	1897	1966
56	995	1031	1067	1105	1144	1185	1227	1271	1316	1362	1411	1461	1513	1566	1622	1679	1739	1801	1864	1931	1999
57	1021	1057	1094	1132	1172	1213	1255	1299	1345	1392	1441	1491	1544	1598	1654	1712	1772	1834	1898	1964	2033
58	1047	1084	1121	1160	1200	1242	1285	1329	1375	1422	1472	1523	1575	1630	1686	1744	1805	1867	1932	1999	2068
59	1074	1111	1149	1188	1229	1271	1314	1359	1406	1454	1503	1555	1608	1663	1719	1778	1839	1902	1966	2034	2103
60	1102	1139	1178	1217	1258	1301	1345	1390	1437	1485	1535	1587	1641	1696	1753	1812	1873	1936	2002	2069	2139
61	1130	1168	1207	1247	1289	1331	1376	1421	1469	1518	1568	1620	1674	1730	1788	1847	1908	1972	2038	2105	2175
62	1160	1198	1237	1278	1319	1363	1408	1454	1501	1551	1602	1654	1709	1765	1823	1882	1944	2008	2074	2142	2212
63	1189	1228	1268	1309	1351	1395	1440	1487	1535	1585	1636	1689	1744	1800	1858	1919	1981	2045	2111	2180	2250
64	1220	1259	1299	1341	1384	1428	1473	1520	1569	1619	1671	1724	1779	1836	1895	1956	2018	2082	2149	2218	2289
65	1251	1291	1332	1373	1417	1461	1507	1555	1604	1655	1707	1760	1816	1873	1932	1993	2056	2121	2188	2256	2328
66	1284	1324	1365	1407	1451	1496	1542	1590	1640	1691	1743	1797	1853	1911	1970	2031	2094	2160	2227	2296	2367
67	1317	1357	1399	1441	1486	1531	1578	1626	1676	1728	1780	1835	1891	1949	2009	2070	2134	2199	2267	2336	2408
68	1351	1391	1433	1477	1521	1567	1615	1663	1713	1765	1819	1873	1930	1988	2048	2110	2174	2240	2307	2377	2449
69	1385	1427	1469	1513	1558	1604	1652	1701	1752	1804	1857	1913	1970	2028	2089	2151	2215	2281	2350	2418	2490
70	1421	1463	1506	1550	1595	1642	1690	1740	1791	1843	1897	1953	2010	2069	2130	2192	2256	2322	2391	2461	2533
71	1458	1500	1543	1588	1633	1681	1729	1779	1830	1883	1938	1994	2051	2110	2171	2234	2299	2365	2433	2504	2576
72	1495	1538	1581	1626	1673	1720	1769	1819	1871	1924	1979	2035	2093	2153	2214	2277	2342	2408	2477	2547	2620
73	1534	1577	1621	1666	1713	1761	1810	1861	1913	1966	2021	2078	2136	2196	2258	2321	2386	2453	2521	2592	2665
74	1573	1616	1661	1707	1754	1802	1852	1903	1955	2009	2065	2122	2180	2240	2302	2365	2431	2498	2566	2637	2710
75	1614	1657	1702	1749	1796	1845	1895	1946	1999	2053	2109	2166	2225	2285	2347	2411	2476	2543	2612	2683	2756
76	1655	1699	1745	1791	1839	1888	1939	1990	2043	2098	2154	2211	2270	2331	2393	2457	2523	2590	2659	2730	2803
77	1698	1742	1788	1835	1883	1933	1983	2035	2089	2144	2200	2258	2317	2378	2440	2504	2570	2638	2707	2778	2851
78	1741	1786	1833	1880	1928	1978	2029	2082	2135	2191	2247	2305	2365	2426	2488	2553	2618	2686	2755	2827	2899
79	1786	1832	1878	1926	1975	2025	2076	2129	2183	2238	2295	2353	2413	2474	2537	2602	2668	2735	2805	2876	2949
80	1832	1878	1925	1973	2022	2073	2124	2177	2232	2287	2344	2403	2463	2524	2587	2652	2718	2785	2855	2926	2999
81	1879	1926	1973	2021	2071	2121	2173	2227	2281	2337	2394	2453	2513	2575	2638	2702	2769	2837	2906	2977	3050
82	1928	1974	2022	2070	2120	2171	2224	2277	2332	2388	2446	2504	2565	2626	2690	2754	2821	2889	2958	3029	3102
83	1978	2024	2072	2121	2171	2223	2275	2329	2384	2440	2498	2557	2617	2679	2743	2807	2874	2942	3011	3082	3155

FL (mm)	Abdominal Circumference (mm)																			
	305	310	315	320	325	330	335	340	345	350	355	360	365	370	375	380	385	390	395	400
40	1590	1658	1729	1802	1879	1959	2042	2129	2220	2314	2413	2515	2622	2734	2850	2972	3098	3230	3367	3511
41	1617	1685	1756	1830	1907	1987	2071	2158	2249	2344	2442	2545	2652	2764	2880	3002	3128	3260	3397	3540
42	1644	1712	1783	1858	1935	2016	2100	2187	2279	2373	2472	2575	2683	2794	2911	3032	3159	3290	3427	3570
43	1671	1740	1812	1886	1964	2045	2129	2217	2308	2404	2503	2606	2713	2825	2942	3063	3189	3321	3458	3600
44	1699	1768	1840	1915	1993	2075	2159	2247	2339	2434	2533	2637	2744	2856	2973	3094	3220	3352	3488	3630
45	1727	1797	1869	1944	2023	2105	2189	2278	2370	2465	2565	2668	2776	2888	3004	3125	3251	3383	3519	3661
46	1756	1826	1898	1974	2053	2135	2220	2309	2401	2497	2596	2700	2807	2919	3036	3157	3283	3414	3550	3692
47	1785	1855	1928	2004	2084	2166	2251	2340	2432	2528	2628	2732	2840	2952	3068	3189	3315	3446	3582	3723
48	1814	1885	1959	2035	2115	2197	2283	2372	2464	2560	2660	2764	2872	2984	3100	3221	3347	3478	3613	3754
49	1845	1916	1990	2066	2146	2229	2315	2404	2497	2593	2693	2797	2905	3017	3133	3254	3380	3510	3645	3786
50	1875	1947	2021	2098	2178	2261	2347	2437	2530	2626	2726	2830	2938	3050	3166	3287	3412	3542	3677	3818
51	1906	1978	2053	2130	2210	2294	2380	2470	2563	2659	2760	2864	2972	3084	3200	3320	3445	3575	3710	3850
52	1938	2010	2085	2163	2243	2327	2413	2503	2597	2693	2794	2898	3006	3117	3234	3354	3479	3608	3743	3882
53	1970	2043	2118	2196	2277	2360	2447	2537	2631	2728	2828	2932	3040	3152	3268	3388	3513	3642	3776	3915
54	2003	2076	2151	2229	2311	2395	2482	2572	2665	2762	2863	2967	3075	3186	3302	3422	3547	3676	3809	3948
55	2036	2109	2185	2264	2345	2429	2516	2607	2700	2797	2898	3002	3110	3221	3337	3457	3581	3710	3843	3981
56	2070	2143	2220	2298	2380	2464	2552	2642	2736	2833	2933	3038	3145	3257	3372	3492	3616	3744	3877	4015
57	2104	2178	2254	2333	2415	2500	2587	2678	2772	2869	2970	3074	3181	3293	3408	3527	3651	3779	3911	4048
58	2139	2213	2290	2369	2451	2536	2624	2714	2808	2905	3006	3110	3218	3329	3444	3563	3686	3814	3946	4082
59	2175	2249	2326	2405	2488	2573	2660	2751	2845	2942	3043	3147	3254	3366	3480	3599	3722	3849	3981	4117
60	2211	2286	2363	2442	2525	2610	2698	2789	2883	2980	3080	3184	3292	3403	3517	3636	3758	3885	4016	4151
61	2248	2323	2400	2480	2562	2647	2736	2827	2921	3018	3118	3222	3329	3440	3554	3673	3795	3921	4052	4186
62	2285	2360	2438	2518	2600	2686	2774	2865	2959	3056	3157	3260	3367	3478	3592	3710	3832	3957	4087	4222
63	2323	2398	2476	2556	2639	2725	2813	2904	2998	3095	3195	3299	3406	3516	3630	3747	3869	3994	4124	4257
64	2362	2437	2515	2595	2678	2764	2852	2943	3037	3134	3235	3338	3445	3555	3668	3785	3906	4031	4160	4293
65	2401	2477	2555	2635	2718	2804	2892	2983	3077	3174	3274	3378	3484	3594	3707	3824	3944	4069	4197	4329
66	2441	2517	2595	2675	2759	2845	2933	3024	3118	3215	3315	3418	3524	3633	3746	3863	3983	4106	4234	4366
67	2481	2557	2636	2716	2800	2885	2974	3065	3159	3256	3355	3458	3564	3673	3786	3902	4021	4144	4271	4402
68	2523	2599	2677	2758	2841	2927	3016	3107	3200	3297	3397	3499	3605	3714	3826	3941	4060	4183	4309	4439
69	2564	2641	2719	2800	2884	2969	3058	3149	3242	3339	3438	3541	3646	3754	3866	3981	4100	4222	4347	4477
70	2607	2683	2762	2843	2927	3012	3101	3192	3285	3381	3481	3583	3688	3796	3907	4022	4140	4261	4386	4514
71	2650	2727	2806	2887	2970	3056	3144	3235	3328	3424	3523	3625	3730	3838	3948	4062	4180	4300	4425	4552
72	2694	2771	2850	2931	3014	3100	3188	3279	3372	3468	3567	3668	3816	3880	3990	4104	4220	4340	4464	4591
73	2739	2816	2895	2976	3059	3145	3233	3323	3416	3512	3610	3712	3816	3922	4032	4145	4261	4381	4503	4629
74	2785	2861	2940	3021	3105	3190	3278	3369	3461	3557	3655	3756	3859	3966	4075	4187	4303	4421	4543	4668
75	2831	2908	2987	3068	3151	3236	3324	3414	3507	3602	3700	3800	3903	4009	4118	4230	4344	4462	4583	4708
76	2878	2955	3034	3115	3198	3283	3371	3461	3553	3648	3745	3845	3948	4053	4161	4272	4387	4504	4624	4747
77	2926	3003	3081	3162	3245	3331	3418	3508	3600	3694	3791	3891	3993	4098	4205	4316	4429	4545	4665	4787
78	2974	3051	3130	3211	3294	3379	3466	3555	3647	3741	3838	3937	4039	4143	4250	4360	4472	4588	4706	4827
79	3024	3100	3179	3260	3343	3427	3514	3604	3695	3789	3885	3984	4085	4188	4295	4404	4515	4630	4748	4868
80	3074	3151	3229	3310	3392	3477	3564	3653	3744	3837	3933	4031	4131	4234	4340	4448	4559	4673	4790	4909
81	3125	3202	3280	3360	3443	3527	3614	3702	3793	3886	3981	4079	4179	4281	4386	4493	4604	4716	4832	4950
82	3177	3253	3332	3412	3494	3578	3664	3752	3843	3935	4030	4127	4226	4328	4432	4539	4648	4760	4875	4992
83	3230	3306	3384	3464	3546	3630	3716	3803	3893	3985	4080	4176	4275	4376	4479	4585	4693	4804	4918	5034

GLOSSARY

Abortion   The loss of a pregnancy before 28 weeks gestation. This may be spontaneous or induced.

Abruption   Separation of the placenta before the third stage of labour.

Absorption   The process by which ultrasound energy is dissipated. Energy is passed to the particles of the medium through which the ultrasound beam is travelling and produces heat.

Acetylcholinesterase   An enzyme found in the amniotic fluid in the presence of a neural tube defect.

Acidosis   A decrease in the blood pH.

Acoustic impedance   The retarding effect that a medium has on the passage of a sound wave.

Acoustic shadow   An area of darkness that occurs behind a highly attenuating structure. For example, the dark area that occurs beneath a directly anterior fetal spine shadowing the umbilical vein.

Acoustic window   A structure that has little or no acoustic impedance and thus allows easy passage of sound and visualisation of deeper structures.

Agenesis   Failure of formation.

Alphafetoprotein   A protein produced by the yolk sac or fetal liver. High levels in the maternal serum or amniotic fluid may indicate a neural tube defect.

Amelia   Absence of a long bone.

Amenorrhoea   Absence of periods.

Amplitude   The maximum difference between the peaks and troughs of an ultrasound wave.

Amplitude (A) mode   A means of displaying echoes such that the amplitude of the echo is represented by the size of the deflection on the vertical axis of the oscilloscope. The distance between two such deflections represents depth (time).

Anechoic   Producing no echoes.

Angioma   A benign tumour of blood vessels.

Angle of asynclitism   The angle between the midline echo from the fetal head and the vertical.

Anteflexed   The forward bending of the body of the uterus on the cervix.

Anteroposterior   Front to back.

Anteverted   Tilted forward.

Artifact   False information.

Ascites   An accumulation of fluid in the abdominal cavity.

Atresia   Congenital absence or closure of a normal body opening or tubular structure.

Attenuation   A decrease in the amplitude of the ultrasound wave due to absorption, scattering, reflection and refraction.

Autosomal recessive   A mode of inheritance which gives the offspring a 1 in 4 chance of having the disease.

Axial resolution   The minimum distance between two points that the ultrasound system is able to discriminate along the axis of the ultrasound beam. This is proportional to the pulse length.

Bandwidth   The range of frequencies contained in an ultrasound pulse. The pulse is usually referred to by the principle frequency only.

Beam   The field that is insonated by the transducer.

Beam steering   An electronic means of focusing an ultrasound beam.

Beam width   The cross-section of the ultrasound beam at a given point.

Benign   Not malignant. Not cancer.

Brachycephaly   A short, wide head.

Brightness (B) mode   A means of displaying echoes such that a spot on the ultrasound screen is in the same relative location as the source of the echoes. Furthermore the brightness of the spot corresponds to the magnitude of the echo.

Calipers   Electronic measuring devices that can be positioned on the screen by the user.

Caudal   Relating to the tail.

Cavum septum pellucidum   A space between the membranes that separate the anterior horns of the lateral cerebral ventricles.

Cephalad   In the direction towards the head.

Cephalopelvic disproportion   A discrepancy between the size of the fetal head and the pelvis.

Cervix   The neck of the uterus.

Chorioangioma   A collection of fetal blood vessels that form a tumour on the placental surface.

Clomiphene   A drug that stimulates ovulation by initiating the natural menstrual cycle.

Coronal plane   The plane that is parallel to the front of the subject, hence it is often called the frontal plane.

Corpus luteum   An endocrine body formed after ovulation from the ruptured ovarian follicle.

Coupling gel   A medium that is a very weak attenuator and whose purpose is to exclude air (a strong attenuator) from between the transducer and the patient.

Craniosynostosis   Premature fusion of the cranial sutures.

Decibel   A notation for measuring sound. It relates one source of sound to another as a ratio and so eliminates the need for absolute measurement.

Decidual reaction   The change that occurs to the endometrium during pregnancy.

Delay   An electronic means of ignoring signals from the near field.

Depth   The distance between the interface being insonated and the front surface of the transducer. It is calculated from the formula: $Depth = velocity \times go\text{-}return\ time/2$ where velocity is the assumed speed of ultrasound in tissue (usually 1540 m/s).

Dextrorotation   Twisted to the right.

Distal   Furthest from the trunk or the origin.

Dizygotic   Developing from two fertilised ova.

Dolichocephaly   A narrow, long head.

Ductus venosus   A fetal vessel that runs through the liver and joins the umbilical vein to the vena cava.

Dynamic range/focusing   A method whereby several waves are used to image the tissue. By the use of a time gate the echoes from each wave are limited so that they give information from a specific tissue depth. The final image is built up from several (usually six) layers.

Dysplasia   Abnormal tissue development.

Dystocia   Difficult childbirth.

Echo   The returning signal from an interface.

Echogenicity   The ability of a medium to return echoes.

Ectopic pregnancy   A pregnancy that implants outside the uterine cavity.

Ectrodactyly   The lobster claw deformity.

Endometrium   The lining of the uterine cavity.

Focal zone   The region of the beam where the resolution is greatest.

Foramen ovale   A connection between the cardiac atria of the fetus that closes at birth.

Frame rate   The number of images displayed per second. If this is greater than 20 a flicker-free image is produced.

Gain   Amplification.

Gamma control   A means of displaying the grey scale such that it is appropriate for the hard copy or the display.

Germinal matrix   The lining of the lateral cerebral ventricles.

Grey scale   A method of displaying the amplitude of the echoes as shades of grey.

Gestational age   The length of pregnancy based upon a reliable LMP, assuming that conception occurs 14 days later.

Hard copy   A permanent record of the image, e.g. Polaroid pictures or videotape.

Hertz   Cycles per second.

Heterozygous   Carrying only one half of the gene pair that causes a disease.

Holoprosencephaly   Failure of cleavage of the prosencephalon (early forebrain) associated with defects in midline facial structures or cyclops.

Homogeneous   Having similar structures.

Homozygous   Carrying both of a gene pair.

Human chorionic gonadotrophin (HCG)   A hormone which is produced by the placenta. Detecting HCG in the blood of a woman is the first sign of pregnancy. HCG is also very similar to LH and is used to mimic the LH surge and so cause ovulation in patients having Pergonal therapy.

Hyaline degeneration   The breakdown of the muscle of a fibroid into an amorphous mass.

Hyperemesis gravidarum   Severe vomiting in early pregnancy.

Hypertension   High blood pressure.

Hypocalcaemia   An abnormally low concentration of calcium in the blood.

Hypoglycaemia   An abnormally low concentration of glucose in the blood.

Hypothermia   A subnormal body temperature.

Hypoxia   A shortage of oxygen.

Insonation   Exposure to the sound beam.

Interface   The boundary between two media (or changes of texture within a medium). The interface will only be echogenic if the acoustic impedances on either side are different.

Internal os   The junction between the cervix and the body of the uterus.

Karyotype   The chromosomal make-up of an individual or a cell line.

L:S ratio   Lecithin:sphingomyelin ratio — a ratio of fatty acids found in the amniotic fluid which helps to determine fetal lung maturity.

Lateral   On one side.

Lateral resolution   The minimum distance that the system is able to discriminate between two points at right angles to the ultrasound beam.

Linear array   A means of producing a real-time image in which there are multiple small piezoelectric crystals in a linear arrangement.

Longitudinal   Running lengthwise, in the direction of the long axis of the body.

Luteinised unruptured follicle (LUF)   The formation of a corpus luteum from an ovarian follicle that has not released its ovum.

Luteinising hormone   A pituitary hormone that is produced in mid-cycle which probably causes ovulation.

Macrosomia   A big baby — usually greater than the 90th centile for gestational age.

Malignant   Cancerous.

Marginal sinus   A large vein that is found at the edge of the placenta.

Mechanical sector scanner   A method of producing real-time images in which two or three transducers are rotated on a central axis.

Medial   Near the centre or middle.

Megahertz (MHz)   Million(s) of cycles per second.

Meromelia   Congenital absence of part but not all of a limb.

Metaphysis   The wider part at the end of the shaft of the long bone.

Micromelia   Congenital shortness of the long bones.

M-mode (T-M mode)   Time-motion mode. A means of displaying echoes such that variations in the A-mode are recorded in the y-axis.

Miscarriage   The lay term for a spontaneous abortion.

Monozygotic   Arising from a single fertilised ovum.

Multiparous   Having had one or more pregnancy.

Myometrium   The smooth muscle coat of the uterus.

Neoplasm   A tumour. May be benign or malignant.

Noise   Unwanted signals that arise from the electronics of the equipment or from random echoes.

Nulliparous   Having had no pregnancies.

Oblique   Slanting or deviating from the longitudinal or transverse.

Occiput   The lower, back part of the head.

Orthogonal   At right angles to.

Ovulation   The release of the ovum from the ovarian follicle.

Paroxysmal   Intermittent.

Pergonal   Human menopausal gonadotrophins. These stimulate the production of ovarian follicles in place of natural pituitary gonadotrophins. Once the follicles have achieved the desired size it is necessary to give HCG to produce ovulation.

Peristalsis   A wave of alternating contraction and relaxation which propels food along the bowel.

Phased array   A method of producing real-time images in which the individual elements of the transducer are excited sequentially so producing a beam that can be steered.

Phocomelia   Congenital absence of the long bones with the hands and feet attached to the trunk by a single short bone.

Piezoelectric effect   The ability to transduce sound waves to an electrical current and vice versa.

Pixel   A picture element.

Placenta circumvallata   A ditch that surrounds the placenta causing the membranes to be inserted a short way from the edge of the placenta.

Pleural effusion   A collection of fluid between the lung and the chest wall.

Polycythaemia   An increase in the red cell mass in the blood.

Posterolateral   Behind and to one side.

Postmenstrual age   The length of pregnancy based upon the LMP irrespective of its reliability.

Pre-eclampsia   A syndrome of hypertension and proteinuria that only occurs in pregnancy.

Preterm   Before 37 completed weeks of pregnancy.

Proteinuria   More than 300 mg/1 of protein in the maternal urine.

Proximal   Nearest to the trunk or the origin.

Pterygium   A wing-like structure, e.g. pterygium coli is a web from the jaw to the shoulder.

Pulmonary hypoplasia   Underdevelopment of the fetal lungs.

Pulse repetition frequency (PRF)   The number of times that an ultrasound pulse is produced per second.

Real-time   A means of displaying serial B-mode images so rapidly that motion appears continuous to the human eye.

Reflection   Alteration of the direction of the ultrasound beam due to an interface which is several times larger than the wavelength of that beam.

Refraction   The bend observed in a sound or light wave when it travels between two media of differing acoustic impedances.

Retroflexed   The backward bending of the uterus on the cervix.

Retroverted   Tilted backwards.

Reverberation   Multiple images between the target and the transducer (or within the target) caused by the echoes being reflected back into the tissue being insonated.

Rhizomelia   Congenital shortening of the proximal long bones, i.e. humerus and femur.

Sacrum   The lower part of the spine.

Scattering   Reflection of ultrasound energy from an interface which is equal to or less than the wavelength of the incident beam.

Sinciput   The upper, front part of the head.

Sinus rhythm   The beating of the heart that occurs in response to an electric stimulus from the sino-atrial node.

Slope   The rate of increase in amplification with depth.

Small for gestational age (small for dates)   Fetal biometry measurements or a birthweight that is small (usually less than the 10th centile) for gestation.

Sonolucent   Producing few echoes.

Static scanner   A system in which two-dimensional images are obtained by movement of a single crystal.

Succenturate lobe   A part of the placenta separated from the main body. It is usually connected by fetal vessels which — if they lie over the cervix — are known as vasa praevia.

Supine hypotension   A fall in blood pressure caused by the pregnant uterus occluding the inferior vena cava and decreasing cardiac output.

Suppression   An electronic means of reducing noise.

Syndactyly   Webbed fingers or toes.

Teratoma   A tumour composed of multiple tissue types not usually found in that area.

Time gain control (TGC)   A means of increasing the amplification of echoes with time (depth) such that echoes from deeper tissues are not lost.

Time-motion (T-M) mode   See M-mode.

TORCH   Toxoplasmosis, rubella, cytomegalovirus, herpes. These are the common infectious agents that affect the fetus.

Transducer   A device (and its housing) composed of one or more piezoelectric crystals that will convert voltages to ultrasound energy and ultrasound to voltages.

Transonic   Allowing sound to pass through it, i.e. a poor attenuator.

Transverse   A plane that is perpendicular to the longitudinal plane. In the case of the fetus this usually means a plane at right angles to the fetal spine.

Trimester   One third of pregnancy.

Triploidy   Having 69 chromosomes.

Ultrasound   Sound with frequencies above the range of human hearing (more than 20 kHz). Diagnostically usable ultrasound is usually in the range of 2–10 MHz.

Vasa praevia   Fetal vessels that overlie the cervix. They arise from a velamentous insertion of the cord or from a succenturate lobe.

***x*-axis (abscissa)**   The horizontal scale of a graph or oscilloscope.

***y*-axis (ordinate)**   The vertical scale of a graph or oscilloscope.

Zygote   A fertilised egg.

FURTHER READING

Basic ultrasound

British Medical Ultrasound Society 1990 Clinical applications of ultrasonic fetal measurements. British Institute of Radiology, London
Jeanty P, Romero R 1984 Obstetrical ultrasound. McGraw-Hill, New York

Advanced ultrasound

Allan L D 1987 Manual of fetal echocardiography. MTP Press
Lilford R 1990 Prenatal diagnosis and prognosis. Butterworths
Pearce J M F 1992 Doppler ultrasound in perinatal medicine. Oxford University Press
Romero R, Pilu G, Jeanty P, Ghidini A, Hobbins J C 1987 Prenatal diagnosis of congenital anomalies. Appleton & Lange, New York
Teague M J et al 1985 A combined ultrasonic linear array scanner and pulsed Doppler velocimeter for the estimation of blood flow in the fetus and the adult abdomen I: Technical aspects. Ultrasound in Medicine and Biology 11:27–36
Whittle M, Connor M J 1989 Prenatal diagnosis. Blackwell

Physics and safety

British Medical Ultrasound Society 1990 Safety of ultrasound report.
McDicken N 1981 Diagnostic ultrasonics: principles and use of instruments, 2nd edn. Wiley, Chichester
National Institute of Health 1984 Diagnostic ultrasound in pregnancy. Consensus statement from Consensus Development Conference
Royal College of Obstetricians and Gynaecologists 1985 Diagnostic ultrasound: biological effects and possible hazards. RCOG Publications, London
Stewart H F, Stratmeyer M E (eds) 1982 An overview of ultrasound theory, measurement, medical application, and biological effects. U.S. Department of Health and Human Services, Food and Drug Administration

INDEX

Multiple pregnancy, 60–63
  abortion, 68
  amniocentesis, 174–5
  determining gestational age, 93, 219
  increased fetal risk, 216–19

Naegele's formula, 77
Neural tube defects, 123, 124–5
  see also Anencephaly; Spina bifida
Noise, 259
Nuchal fat pad, 167–9, Appendix Three

Obstructive uropathy, 148–52
Obturator internus muscle, 30, 32
Occipitofrontal diameter, 85
Oesophageal atresia, 140
Oligohydramnios, 146
  causes, 288
  Doppler ultrasound, 234–5
Omphalocoele, 141–2, 290
On-screen measurement, 7
Operators, 9–10
Osteogenesis imperfecta, 155
Ovaries
  abdominal scanning, 28–33
  cancer, 34–5
  cysts, 35–6
    multiple (hyperstimulation syndrome), 42
    in pregnancy, 37
  follicles, 34
    cysts, 35, 37
    luteinised unruptured follicle syndrome, 40–41
    monitoring development, 37–43
  malignancy, 34–5
  masses, 35–7
  measurement, 33–5
  in Pouch of Douglas, 29
  transvaginal scanning, 33
Ovulation
  induced, 41–2
  monitoring, 37–43

Patients, preparation, 8–9
Pelvi-ureteric junction obstruction (PUJO), 148–51
Pelvis, normal, 14–43
Percutaneous umbilical blood sampling (PUBS; cordocentesis), 176–9
Pergonal, 41
Phased array transducers, 262–3
Phocomelia, 152
Placenta, 53–5, 186–99
  abruption, 194–7, 215
  chorioangioma, 198
  circumvallata, 197–8

Placenta (contd)
  cysts, 193
  grading, 193
  insufficiency, 202, 234, 235
  lakes, 192
  locating in early pregnancy, 186–8
  malignancy, 198
  marginal sinus bleed, 198
  praevia, 187, 188–91
Polaroid photographs, 7–8
Polycystic kidney disease, infantile, 146–7
Polydactyly, 156
Polyhydramnios, 138
  causes, 288
Porencephalic cysts, 134–5
Portal veins, 111
Post-processing (gamma correction), 264–5
Posterior fossa, 99
  abnormalities, 135
Posterior horn: cerebral hemisphere ratio (PVHR), 97–8, 128
Posterior urethral valves, 151–2
Postmenstrual age, 77
Pouch of Douglas, ovaries in, 29
Pre-processing, 5, 263
Pregnancy
  abortion, 64–8
  anembryonic, 64–5
  bleeding, causes, 287
  early, 44–63
    amniocentesis, 171–4
    complications, 64–76
    locating the placenta, 186–8
  ectopic, 68–73
  failure (abortion), 64–8
  fibroids, 24–5
  heterotopic, 69
  implantation bleed, 53–5
  late, 214–21
  marginal sinus bleed, 198
    amniocentesis, 175–6
  multiple, 60–63
  ovarian masses, 37
  tests, and ectopic gestation, 69
  transvaginal scanning, 44
  twin see Twin pregnancy
Premature rupture of membranes (PROM), 235
  amniocentesis, 176
Presentation, fetal, 219–20
  breech see Breech presentation
  transverse, 81–2
Preterm labour, 215
Probes, 1–4, 253–8, 261–3
  abdominal, movements, 10–12
  movements, 10–13
  transvaginal, 9
    movements, 12–13
Proboscis, 166